THIRD FLOOR SUMMER

A MOTHER'S MEMOIR OF HER JOURNEY BATTLING CANCER

MARA SOLOMON

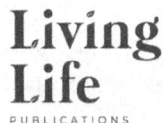

Living
Life
PUBLICATIONS

Third Floor Summer: A Mother's Memoir of Her Journey Battling Cancer

Cover by Madelyn Copperwaite, MC Creative LLC
First edition, October 2024
ISBN: 979-8-218-49434-6
Library of Congress Control Number: 2024917292
Created in the United States of America

Learn more about Mara Solomon at LivingLifeAfterCancer.com. Special discounts are available on quantity book purchases. Contact Mara Solomon at Mara@LivingLife-AfterCancer.com for more information.

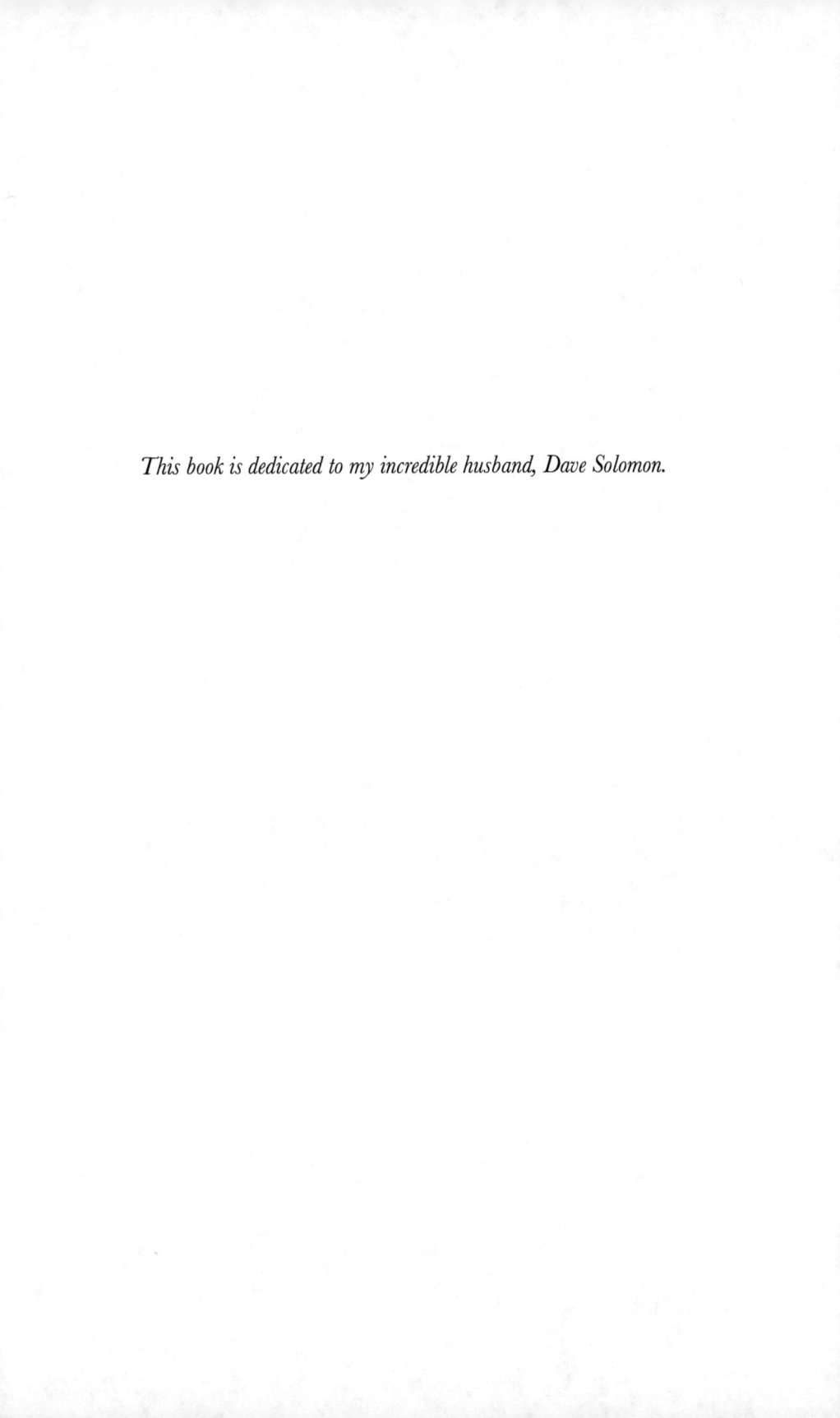

This book is dedicated to my incredible husband, Dave Solomon.

INTRODUCTION

My cell phone rang as I walked home from the store with the kids. It was my parents, so of course I answered it; I can't ignore them. We talk every morning. I love catching up with them to let the kids hear their voices and vice versa. I accepted the call with my usual upbeat and happy, "Hello." It was my mom, and there was something unusual in the way she responded to me. There was no "Good Morning" or "How are you?" She sternly said, "We reviewed the labs you sent over last night and spoke to our oncologist friend. We are on our way to your house. You need to get home, get in the car, and have Dave take you to the ER immediately."

Little would I know how important that phone call was.

LET ME TELL YOU A LITTLE ABOUT ME...

I don't want to brag, but I will. I have an amazing life. I have a great husband; we have been married 6 and a half years and throughout that time we have made the most of our marriage. We've done everything right. We bought a house in the suburbs, got a dog and we now have 2 great kids. Our daughters are ages 4 and 1. I really am living the dream. This is everything I ever wanted.

It hasn't been easy to get all of that. With both of us working full time, our kids are in day care Monday through Friday. This means I must have a well-scheduled day that goes like this: waking up early, make breakfast, get kids' meals packed for school, take them to day care/ preschool, off to work, then a day full of work, drive home in traffic, get the kids from day care, go home, play with the kids, make dinner, bedtime routine with the kids then maybe have an hour with Dave and then off to sleep. The great thing about being married is that I get to share all of the at home tasks with Dave. I cannot imagine if I didn't have him (ooh aah). When it comes to bedtime, I often fall asleep nursing my 1-year-old to sleep. Yes, my little one still nurses. Not only does she nurse to sleep, she also wakes up at about 2 each morning needing to nurse again. I know what you are thinking. why doesn't your 1-year-old stop nursing, but for some reason she is not ready. Okay, really, I'm not ready for her to stop, but don't judge me for that.

I loved our schedule, and after Eli was born, I decided it was really important that I make sure I add a little me time into that schedule. You know how the flight attendants say to put your oxygen masks on first before helping others. Those words of wisdom became one of my life mottos. I created a daily routine that did exactly that. I decided that if I was not at my best, then how could I be my best for others? I started an exercise routine where I went to the gym at 5 a.m. multiple days a week, I ate a healthy breakfast, and continued our great scheduled day. Everyone saw me being healthy and honestly, it would make you nauseated how I had my healthy routine down to a science.

We lived the healthiest life. Or did we?

With the kids in daycare and preschool, it was inevitable they would bring home a cold of some sort, and of course they would share it with us. 2013 was a tough year. The whole family got to share several colds, the stomach flu, and even got lice. Lucky us! As summer approached, it seemed unseasonal, but I accepted that it was okay to be feeling these flu-like symptoms again. I had come to expect them.

Since earlier this month, I had been feeling a mixture of flu-like symptoms, a low-grade fever for a month, a slight cough, a bit of nausea (paired with panic feelings... oh gosh, I hope I'm not pregnant... two kids were all that we wanted), hot flashes, and exhaustion. But shoot... I had two young kids, worked full time, and was burning the candle at both ends. It was expected to be tired, right? I also was up a lot of the night, thanks to the middle of the night nursing and getting up early.

In additional to those flu symptoms, I also noticed occasional night sweats and an odd rash but nothing out of the ordinary. The rash wasn't really weird because, did I mention I'm full of freckles? My Irish genes left me with extremely pale skin and lots—I mean lots—of freckles, so a rash made up of tiny red dots on my inner left thigh could really just be a new pattern of freckles. This time it was different from my millions of light brown spots peppered throughout my body. These "freckles" stood out because they consisted of roughly 20 tiny bright red spots making a circle type shape on my inner left thigh. These didn't look like my other freckles. There was something odd about these. What could it be?

Since it was the beginning of summer break, Dave had taken the kids away for a couple days, making it a perfect time for me to schedule an annual check-up with my primary care physician. Life had gotten the best of me, and I had not prioritized this necessary annual appointment. Since taking care of myself was top on my agenda, I wasn't going to put this appointment off anymore.

I compiled a list of concerns that I mentioned above and brought them to my appointment I was ready for the doctor to say: "Well Mara, you have two kids, work full time, are getting up at the crack of dawn to work out, you need to take it easy." I was confident my doctor would brush off the concerns about my smattering of freckles with the rationale that my chaotic life was the root cause of my oddities. Nothing more.

I was very "lucky," a term I have become a frequent user of. We had recently changed insurance, which meant I had never met my primary care physician. I was able to get a last-minute appointment for that day. I was confident the doctor would evaluate my symptoms and encourage me to take it easy. That would be that. I showed up the next day, and for the most part, my appointment ran how I expected. She listened to my concerns and gave me some advice to create more time for me in my life. In addition, she ordered lab work too. I didn't think anything about it.

The blood work included all the basics: the white blood cells (WBC), red blood cells (RBC), neutrophils, and more. I was able to walk down the hall and get my blood taken right then and there. What a convenience! They also told me I would be able to see my results that evening. I've never experienced that. Usually the results are completed, sent to your doctor and you are contacted once your doctor receives them. This being a Friday that would mean I wouldn't know anything until at least Monday. How cool that I could have an idea of what was going on possibly Friday night.

After my labs got drawn, I went home to greet Dave and the kids as soon as they came back from their trip. I was so excited to hear all about their fun night away. Oh, I had missed them so much! We are never away from each other. After the hugs and stories, we put the kids to bed and went to bed at our "crazy late" night bedtime of 10 p.m. For some reason, I couldn't fall asleep. I really tried, but sleep eluded me. I decided to get up and get on the computer. When I opened up my computer, there it was, front and center. An email announcing that my lab results were ready. I couldn't believe it; the results were already there. I sat down and couldn't wait to see what they said. Who knows, I bet my White Blood count was high because I knew I was fighting off something, and that is always indicated by a high WBC.

I opened up the test results and clicked on today's tests. I had never looked at test results online before, but this seemed pretty basic. First, I clicked on WBC. The way they posted my results was really neat. on top it said. WBC Count. Then below it says normal range 3.7-11.1 K/uL. Um... okay that means nothing to me. Here is the cool part. Below that was a long line with yellow on each end and the standard range was green. As I looked for where my numbers were, I saw an arrow on top pointing towards the yellow region below the normal range showing that I was below the normal. I was not expecting that. What does that mean?

I looked through each of my test results, everything from hemoglobin to neutrophils and a bunch of other things that I didn't understand and in every one I was either above or below the standard green line. Shoot, I thought. I didn't expect to be so out of range. This is odd. What does that mean?

I took a deep breath and opted to ignore it, knowing my doctor would follow-up on Monday to tell me what to do next. Off to the couch I went to attempt to fall asleep. I continued to toss and turn and couldn't sleep. I had more hot sweats while on the couch and couldn't get comfortable. I wanted to know what the out-of-range numbers really meant. Why are they so out of standard range? With those questions, I did what any "smart" person would: I went to Google and typed in red spots and low neutrophils. I'd be my own doctor, I thought. Let me tell you from experience, this is bad… yes, a really bad… idea. Don't do it. Even if you are perfectly healthy, which I was confident I was. A Google diagnosis is not a diagnosis you want, especially at 11 p.m. on a Friday night.

Dr. Google offered several potential diagnoses, the major being blood diseases like anemia, leukemia, lymphoma, other blood diseases. What the heck?! There was no way. Why would I have some kind of blood disease? I was sure that there was something wrong with Dr. Google's diagnosis.

I had to reach out to someone to figure out what these labs could mean. Dave was asleep, and he had just been with the kids for the last few days, so I didn't want to wake him up. I then thought I could reach out to my parents. I knew it is the middle of the night, but they told me I could always reach out to them whenever I need anything. Well, I really needed them now. They are both in the medical field, and I knew that they would be able to calm my fears before Monday. I took screenshots of all of my labs and texted them over. I knew they would check them after they woke up. After doing all I could do I tried, yet again, to go to sleep with the confidence I would have more answers in the morning. At least my parents would calm me down.

As the evening went on, I was able to finally get to sleep just in time for my 1-year-old to wake up for her middle of the night breastfeeding. After a few more hours of sleep, we got up for a nice breakfast before the kids and I all got dressed and in the stroller for a quick walk to the local art store. They were hosting a fun kids project with a 4th of July theme. I loved that all the art mess would be contained to a room in the store and not my house. There was going to be water, scissors, glue, pens, and glitter. Oh, anything with kids and glitter should not be done in my house. I also expected this project to last 30-60 minutes. It would allow Dave to enjoy a quiet house and to be on his own. Once we got there and settled down, each kid chose their own 4th of July themed project to do. They cut them, glued them, and poured glitter all over them, and after no more than 10 minutes they were done with the project and ready to leave. We packed up and headed home. So much for my plan of a morning full of activities.

When we were half way home, my phone rang, and my life has never been the same.

That was the call from my parents.

My mom told me to head home immediately, I heard her and even though I heard her clearly all of the words were mumbled together. I picked up the pace and walked those last few blocks to my house faster than I ever had before. I put a smile on my face trying not to show the kids the fear that was building up inside of me. My mind raced with possible reasons as to why she was telling me to go to the ER, why she and my dad were coming over to take care of the kids. This didn't make sense.

I picked up my pace as I kept walking home. I started to put her words together. Something must be seriously wrong. They must have looked at the lab results I sent them. The lab results must have been concerning enough that they reached out to their oncologist friend to get his opinion. If they reached out to him on a Saturday something must be really wrong. Everything was running through my mind. I just keep thinking, how could this be happening? I am so healthy. I have done everything right. I worked out. I ate well. I worked hard. I was trying to be a good mom and good wife. Everything was going the right way; how could everything be falling apart. My mind was spinning around in circles. Oh my goodness. NOOOO. I had to pull it together, I thought. For my kids. For my husband. For me. It was going to be okay; I was going to be okay; everything was going to be okay.

My daughter looked up and asked, "Mommy, is everything okay?"

"Of course, Alyssa. Everything is okay," I responded. "Papa and Grandma are going to come over while Dad and I are going to go on a date."

Sure a "date," that is what we will call it. We hadn't been able to go on a date in a long time with the kids being so young. Is this really what it took? One of us being so sick that we had to go to the ER. The ER is going to be our date?

I felt tears well up in my eyes. Was this really happening to me? To us? Dave met me at the door in shock. We got the kids out of the stroller and grabbed each other in a panic. What was happening? We really had no idea of what was going on and we were in no way prepared for what would come next. My parents had called him to share that they were on their way to the house. While we waited for them, I grabbed what we needed to go to the ER. I'd never been to the hospital before and hadn't a clue what I should pack. The only times I'd been to the hospital was to have my children, but those times I was prepared. For my first child I was induced, so I had plenty of time to prepare. Shoot… I had an overnight bag all packed with cute maternity jammies and everything. But not this time. No one prepared you for what to pack for a trip to the ER. I assumed I should bring a book, my phone, and some snacks since I love to eat, and I assume they don't have food in the ER. Boredom and hunger were two feelings I didn't want to experience in a packed ER waiting room. I had heard stories of people waiting a long time to see a doctor there. I might as well bring things to entertain myself.

As much as I was concerned about the ER visit, I was equally as worried about the kids and how they would navigate their day with this wrinkle in it. I wanted to ensure that they had everything they needed, too. I knew my parents would keep them well fed, but how was Eli going to get her bottles throughout the day if I wasn't there to nurse her. We had birthday parties to attend that day, but we'd have to cancel those. Our whole Saturday was thrown out of whack. I took a deep breath and reminded myself that in the midst of long waits, I could get everything back to order, cleaning up the chaos we were experiencing unexpectedly. I was in panic mode trying to feel like I was in charge of everything when really, I was the most out of control that I had ever been.

When we arrived at the ER triage, I was quickly put in a private room. I was shocked as I had expected a long delay in the waiting room, but today was my lucky day, I guess. Maybe I was back to having luck on my side. Once we got into the room, we just waited for what seemed like the longest hour of my life. Dave and I didn't know what to say to each other. The labs must have shown something but what? Why was nobody saying anything to us? We really had no idea what to expect; we just wanted quick answers so we could take the next steps.

We were instantly calmed when we saw a familiar face. The nurse assigned to me was our friend, Micah, whom we had known for several years. We had children the same age, and I had just seen him the night before at a friend's party. What a lovely diversion from all of our fear. We were able to jump into a friendly conversation. Seeing Micah felt like everything was going to be okay.

Dave and I spent about five hours in the ER as they ran more tests, getting blood work done for every possible thing out there including any possible virus, HIV, hepatitis, parvo, and more. I had to tell my symptoms to over fifteen medical professionals. Around 6:30 p.m. that evening, I was ordered for a chest X-ray and then admitted to the hospital. What the heck? I had never even thought that I would be doing anything other than a few hours, maybe even a full day in the ER. Why was I now being admitted to the hospital? What is going on?

I had expected to be home with my kiddos that evening. I was going to do our bedtime routine. Read books, cuddle, and kiss them good night. Apparently, there was another plan for me tonight. I started to realize that something real was happening. They pulled up the side railings on the gurney that I had already been lounging on all day, unlocked the wheels, and pushed me through the hospital halls, into the elevator and pushed the button to the third floor. I didn't know it then, but I know it now. The third floor of this hospital was my permanent residence for the summer.

When they opened the doors to the room, it was dinner time at the hospital, and I was starving. Even though I had brought some snacks with me for what I thought was a couple hours at the hospital, I hadn't gotten a chance to eat them, and even though I was starving, they didn't look good. I had missed the hospital's scheduled dinner time (which was actually a good thing since hospital food leaves much to be desired). Lucky for us a pizza place we had been wanting to try happened to be right across the street from the hospital. In a sea of fear and concern, we found a silver lining and clung to it with all that we had. Dave went over and grabbed us a delicious pizza dinner. This pizza place (which is now one of our favorites) was one of the good things amongst this awful situation.

Since Dave and I were on our date longer than planned, my parents stayed with the kids for the night and Dave stayed by my side. I needed him more than I knew. Thanks to technology, we were able to FaceTime with the kids. Eli's communication consisted of constantly waving at the camera and Alyssa was a chatterbox. The first thing she said, though, was: "Hey mom, why aren't your eyes open?" We all laughed, and, for the record, my eyes were open, they were just very swollen from a day full of crying.

Once I realized that this room was going to be mine for at least a night, I tried to take a look around and really see what I was dealing with. I don't know the exact size of this room but saying it was 20' by 20' is generous.

Let me tell you about this teeny (but private) room. Once they locked my bed into place I looked to my left and saw that on the wall there was a computer affixed against the wall with a floating keyboard. This was the station where the nurses and doctors stood when they entered my room. There was also a hook where the blood pressure cuff, thermometer, and O2 finger monitor hung. They used these between every nurse shift.

Then there was my small hospital-size bed that had railings on either size to keep me in safely. It felt like an adult crib, but the side railings were lower. I did enjoy that the bed could be lifted and lowered; a pricey feature that people pay big bucks for at home. This came standard in these beds. Behind the bed were a multitude of buttons, knobs, plugs, and controllers to contact people and provide necessities such as oxygen. There was also a controller attached to the wall on a cord that hung onto the bed. This controller allowed me to use the television and also call the nurses for help. Pressing it made a light outside the door turn on, and you could speak to someone at the nurse's station.

Since my diagnosis wasn't solidified yet, the nurses also put a bed alarm on my bed, which required me to call every time I wanted to get out of bed, including when I had to go to the bathroom. Can you imagine what it would be like if every time you moved, a funny alarm would go off? This meant that every time I wanted to do ANYTHING, move out of the bed, go to the bathroom, sit in the chair, wash my hands, get a sip of water or something to eat (you get the point), I had to press a button and wait for someone to hear the alarm or see the light, answer your call, come into your room, turn off the bed alarm and help you to get out of bed to complete the do anything I wanted or needed to do. This drove me nuts, especially since I am an independent woman!

The room also had a single nightstand with a phone resting comfortably on top of it. During my stay in that room, the phone would randomly ring. By the time I finally answered it, if there was a person on the other end, it was usually a wrong number. I'm not sure the purpose of that phone.

As I sat in bed and looked to the right, there were beautiful branches of a big tree. Although the trees made the small room dark, it also made something nice to look out to. It made me think of the movie *Pollyanna*. I used to love watching that movie growing up. Do you remember that beautiful tree she climbed up to the attic and fell out of? Well, I don't plan on climbing this tree, but the branches are beautiful and nice to look at.

Just past the window I see the single chair stuffed into the corner. This is the only place to sit on for my visitors. Or if I ever want to sit anywhere other than the bed, I can sit on it. Now remember getting out of bed sets off an alarm so I am not sure how frequently I will be moving into the chair, but at least it is an option. To the left was a tiny closet to store my belongings. In the final space on the wall, yes there is an itty bit of space left, next to the closet was a washing station for the medical professionals and others to clean up when they visited. The washing station included a sink operated by foot petals for hot and cold water along with an automatic soap machine mounted to the wall above the sink. There was an automatic paper towel machine there also. In the sink I could wash my face, brush my teeth, and store all of my toiletries. Imagine sharing your sink with fifty or so people a day. Fun, right?!

Near the sink were boxes of gloves of different sizes. Although the gloves were for the medical staff, there were times throughout my stay that the kids would blow them up and use them as toy balloons and other imaginary things. Who knew they could be used for so many things?

As if this wasn't enough, stuffed into this small room, there was also a tiny bathroom which included a toilet and a small shower. Are you noticing a theme here? Yes, everything was small. I know I am very lucky (there is that word again) because I didn't have to share a room with another person. The bathroom didn't have a sink because remember, I had a wash station to use for, well everything you would need a sink for. It is amazing how much you use a sink for. That sums up the room and I am happy to say that fortunately, that was the smallest of the hospital rooms that they have on this floor.

As I tried to get settled, I was inundated with nurse after nurse and doctor after doctor. So many questions asked and vitals taken: blood pressure, temperature, weight, diet, drug use, alcohol consumption, safety of my relationship. As each question was asked, my head felt like it was spinning more. What was happening to me? Why was I here? What was going on? Were my kids, okay? Why was I going to spend the night here and not at home? Who was going to nurse my baby? I had so many questions and so few answers.

The path to knowledge required more blood tests. I learned that to find a diagnosis required us to rule out as many possible diagnoses as we could. As we checked off potential diagnoses, the doctors leaned more and more toward the worst-case scenario. They decided to schedule a bone marrow biopsy, which is what would provide the most definitive answers.

Warning this paragraph describes a medical procedure, so if you think it will gross you out skip to the next paragraph.

To perform the bone marrow biopsy, it required both a doctor and a nurse to be present. First, I laid down on my stomach and they pulled my pants down to my hips so they could pull the marrow from (the medical term) the posterior iliac crest. Or as I like to call it, the back of my hip bone. They cleaned the area using an iodine covered sponge and then covered everything other than a 3" by 3" square over the bone. Using a syringe filled with lidocaine, they poked the needle through the skin all of the way to the bone and began delivering lidocaine to numb the area. The initial pinch or sting as the needle went into the skin was the most painful part of the procedure. They waited a minute or 2 for the lidocaine to kick in. At this point I wasn't feeling anything. Then the doctor pulled out the bone marrow aspiration tool. I'm sure it has a proper name, but that doesn't matter. It looks like a hollow T shaped awl that is pushed through the skin into and through the bone. I could feel that the doctor had hit the bone because he started really pushing with pressure. I mean he had to get through the external part of the bone into the inner spongy part of the bone. Once he got into the bone, he looked to do two things. To get the aspiration or the liquid part of the marrow and a piece of bone. By using a syringe he sucked the marrow from within the bone. You know how I said the most painful part of this process was the initial lidocaine shot. Well that is true. This didn't hurt at all. The best way I can describe it is it felt like something was being sucked out of my bone. It didn't feel good or bad, just strange. After the doctor got enough liquid bone marrow from the aspiration, he wanted to take out a sliver of bone. This piece of the bone was approximately an inch in length and a millimeter or so in diameter. The great thing about this was that although it sounded gross and painful, it really wasn't. Once they pulled it out, they then taped a piece of gauze on a needle-sized hole in my back and put a big piece of tape over it. Then they asked me to lay on my back to apply pressure on it. The only pain I felt was similar to a bruise for the next couple days. Then they put the bone specimen and liquid on a collection plate. It was really neat to look at. The outside bone was hard, and the inner part looked spongy.

Okay, if you stepped away to avoid reading the medical procedure stuff, you can come back now.

The results from this gave us the information needed to figure out what we were dealing with. In my mind the worst possible diagnosis would be leukemia. Dr. Google had already placed its possibility in my thoughts, but I refused to accept it. Other options could be an autoimmune disease or even parvo. I thought parvo was a disease only dogs could have. We have a five-year-old dog, but he has been vaccinated for parvo. It sounds odd, but I wish it is parvo. That is an easily curable disease. Maybe that is all I have. Wouldn't that have been great?

The bone marrow biopsy will take several days for the results to come back. In the meantime, I was being treated with occasional blood transfusions and new platelets when needed to keep me stable while they figured what was going on. I had to accept that my one-night hospital stay would be at least a few days. I guess one positive to being neutropenic (having a low immune system) was that I couldn't be exposed to anyone else, so I got to have a single room, a small room, but I'd take it. To make my daily infusions of saline and other meds acceptable, I was connected to an IV pole, which was attached to me 24/7.

What is ironic about these infusions is that ever since I turned 18, I had donated blood as frequently as every six weeks. I'm not aware of many other kids who looked forward to their 18th birthday so they could donate blood. There I was. The first thing I did when I turned 18 was go to the local red cross and donate blood. I continued to do that routinely for the next 16 years. How ironic, I thought, that something I had done to help others was now something I was the recipient of. Alanis Morrissette should include that in her next song.

A part of my accepting that the hospital would be my new temporary home was the realization that I needed some new clothing. The hospital clothing was not going to cut it. Did they really want me to wear a gown that was open in the back showing everyone my hiney and awful socks with sticky rubber bottoms to make sure I didn't slip on the floor? No way! I learned there were very few things I could control, but clothing was something I could. I understood hospital staff needed to have easy access to all of my cords, but there had to be a better option than those gowns. While fashion had never been my thing, I knew a wardrobe change would do this body and mind some good. At my request (or demand), Dave went home and grabbed some clothes for me to wear so I could at least have daily wardrobe changes and a sense of normalcy.

Get this, remember how I donated blood frequently in the past. Well to "pay me" for my generous donations, I received a not so classy T-shirt which happened to be on the dresser, and easy for Dave to grab when he packed a bag for me. When I opened up the bag of clothes he brought for me, it included the T-shirt that said, I Bleed Red and Gold in 49ers colors, showing my support for the San Francisco 49ers. I laughed. How funny is that? Here I was needing to receive blood transfusions, and I'd be wearing that shirt. Not only did that shirt get us laughing at this awful time, but it helped improve my outfit and get me out of those terrible hospital gowns.

In the days while I waited to hear what was going on with me, I was comforted by visits from my parents, friends, Dave and the kids. Since it was summer, people were more available to visit me. Really the kids were the best. They had no idea what was going on, and all they worried about was their concerns at the moment. The good and bad of having young children is it is easy to be distracted and focus on other things than the potential bad. They also could more easily just go with the flow. They really helped keep me going.

When I realized my health issue was more than a cold, I began a journal. Here are my entries from those first few days.

SUNDAY, JUNE 30, 2013

In the middle of the night, my head was really hurting on the left side. They took me down for a second CT because earlier the CT hadn't focused on the sinuses. This time they wanted to see if I had a sinus infection. Sure enough, it was just on the left side, but this was able to confirm that. Now on top of the saline, they will add in a medication to help mitigate the sinus infection.

The kids got to come visit, and in trying to make this as comfortable of an environment as I can for Alyssa, when she wanted to come into the bathroom with me, I didn't even hesitate. Of course I let her join me. I explained to her how I pee in something called a hat so they can measure my pee, and they empty it when it is full. I also talked to her about all that was going on. She had questions about other bodily functions, and I tried to be very open with her when answering. When I was done and had passed the interrogation, she had to go to the bathroom. I said no big deal, emptied the hat and went to put her on the toilet. She said to me: "Um mom. I would like some privacy here. I am going to the bathroom." Oh, of course, privacy what is that.

The rest of the day continued to be an emotional train wreck, knowing what could be and also being scared of the unknown. Not feeling well and being alone makes it difficult to not freak out about the future, as well as what all of this could potentially mean for our family in the near and far future.

TUESDAY, JULY 2, 2013

This morning Dr. S, my oncologist said that the preliminary results came back from the bone marrow biopsy with exactly the information we DID NOT want. I don't know why I kept hoping or even thinking it could possibly be something else, but I did. We later learned it is Acute Myeloid Leukemia (AML) without additional specification. This then started the ball rolling on procedures that I needed to have done before we started chemo immediately.

The first scan was called a MUGGA Scan. This was interesting. I was taken to the basement in a darkish room with a huge scanner. They took a vial of blood out of my arm IV, and then labeled it along with labeling me. They took that blood to another room for about 15 minutes where they put radiation into the blood. Then they brought the blood back, double checked it with another technician to make sure they gave me back the proper blood (I also was the only patient, so the chance of them mixing up the blood was pretty slim). Then they put the blood back into me. They took an eight-minute video of my heart with the radiated blood. They actually took two separate videos to monitor how my heart is working overall, and they will continue to do this every three months to monitor how my heart reacts after the chemo, which really can wear out my body. The most challenging thing about the whole ordeal was it took about an hour and a half. (Dave actually ran some errands while I was doing this just so he didn't have to sit around waiting.) Meanwhile there was no music in the room. It was a quiet dark room, and although I was able to talk to the technician a bit about him and his life (I just desperately needed a distraction) so I pretty much just cried the whole time thinking again about what potentially could come. I told the guy that next time we need to have music down there because this silence is not going to fly for me.

WEDNESDAY, JULY 3, 2023

More final results came back with more information obviously confirming the previous results. Before there were 18% leukemic cells in my bone marrow; now it is 40% leukemic.

Today was another day filled with emotion and again attempting to grapple with a diagnosis that I never imagined I would ever have to deal with and certainly not right now. Funny that when receiving this diagnosis and the initial chemo plan, I didn't know what questions to ask. This was all a foreign language to me. I grew up with a medical family, but all of these chemo terms were so unknown. The one main concern I had when I asked my doctor was, "Am I going to lose my hair?" Isn't this odd? Here I've been diagnosed with a life-ending disease, and I am worried about my hair. But this is what is important to me. I recall only weeks earlier getting my hair cut, new bangs. I was the thinnest, healthiest or so I thought then I'd ever been. I looked good. Now I am going to lose my hair is my main concern. It makes sense right? My hair is my identity. What was going to happen when it was gone? Here I received more bad news along with my cancer diagnosis. Yes, it was definite. This course of treatment was going to cause me to lose my hair. In addition, this was the treatment I needed to do. For the type of cancer I had, this is what would kill the cancer.

My platelets were extremely low today, so they got me platelets and began to administer them just before they sent me down to the basement where they were going to put in a central line. Apparently due to my situation I am receiving a line called a Gershawn which is an external line. Many cancer patients get a port line that is internal and can be accessed by a needle to draw blood and deliver chemotherapy. Unfortunately, due to my high risk of infection and need to have constant fluid, chemo, and other fluids put into me. I require an external line called a Gershawn to be surgically implanted.

As I got downstairs, I had to sit in a waiting area where they took my temperature, which was 98 degrees upstairs but was 101 and 102 while I was downstairs. This was a bit odd and potentially could have put off the procedure, but due to the urgency to get things started Dr. S asked the surgical team to move forward and start the procedure. The doctor/surgeon was Dr. Young who has a daughter named Mara, but he pronounces it with a more Italian accent. Having this conversation helped calm me down and made me feel more comfortable as I let him, and his team do something that terrified me. The basement crew was interesting. I'm sure if I was in a basement all day, I would be a bit different too, but they have an odd yet fun (possibly slightly inappropriate in front of patients) style of humor. Clearly there were some issues between some of the techs as there were some real passive aggressive statements (again amongst all of this bizarre situation I'm looking for some normalcy).

After 45 minutes or so they took me into a surgical room where again I laid on a massive imaging machine. The amount of radiation I'm around is out of control, but I guess this is par for the course. There was a team of roughly 5 or 6 people there. The guys had the X-ray protectors wrapped around their waists. They were laying out all of the tools on a huge separate table. I almost felt like I was in an episode of the movie *Saw*. It was a bit overwhelming. Again, the inappropriate jokes amongst themselves continued. They gave me a sedative which I was surprised how quickly it took over.

Next thing I know I want to have a conversation but feel like I'm out of it and not in on the overall conversation. I also had some weird feeling like I had been dreaming about Muppets. Do you know that show from the 80s? According to my dream, I was part of the show. Then the procedure was done.

They wheeled me away and back to my room where I got settled again. I was able to see what they did during my surgery downstairs. As I looked down my chest below my collar bone and on top of my chest plate there were two plastic chords dangling out of my chest. I had been told what they were going to be doing but didn't really know. As the anesthesia began to wear off, it felt painful to move my arm forward and back. These new lines dangling out of my chest will be the new ways that they will be delivering chemo, saline and other medications, and drawing blood. One benefit of this is they won't need my IV or picking me anymore.

As I was getting settled, Dave came back to hang out with me. We continued to try to get a hand on what we need to do to get through this. We are so overwhelmed. Everything seems so unreal and unbelievable.

THURSDAY, JULY 4, 2013

Well this is not how we had planned today. I often look forward to the Fourth of July. Our great city hosts an incredible parade that we can walk to from our house. We love inviting people from other cities to come enjoy it with us was so fortunate that Dave, the kids, and our friends came to visit me. Again, this is not how any of us expected to celebrate our country's birthday. There actually was little to no celebration today. Fortunately, the kids really had no idea of what was going on, what was to come in our future. Again, to them I was just in a hotel that they could visit, and I couldn't leave. It was odd but nothing too strange. Hey, we were a crazy family! We were always doing a lot of things different from other families, so this was just our normal, right?

Now that we knew my diagnosis it was full steam ahead. Today I started my first dose of chemotherapy. A woman named Toni Crotti (now Toni Love) came by and did Jin Shin Jytsu to get my body prepared and hopefully reduce any side effects I would be experiencing from chemo. Jin Shin Jytsu is an ancient art of balancing the body's energy. The practitioner (Toni) uses her hands in different parts of my body to allow energy to flow through my body better through treatment. I had learned about this and felt that with all of the chemo and other western medicines that were going to be poisoning my body I wanted to try this. It can't hurt to try this and really with so much going on and so many things that are going on out of my control, I think this is a great thing that I can control. I will probably do this a couple times a week during treatment. I will have to see how I feel if it is helping me.

Later in the day, the chemo started. The first one was called Idaru-bicin. It was delivered over the course of fifteen minutes through a syringe directly into my central line. It felt bizarre, I sat there with the nurse slowly pushing this bright red liquid into my body. She was covered in a gown covering her full body, a mask over her face and gloves on each of her hands to protect her from this poison while she pushed it directly into my bloodstream. Doesn't that seem odd? She is protecting herself externally while they are shooting this poison directly into my bloodstream. After that, they attached my line to a big bag of a chemo called Cytarabine which was 550 ml delivered over twenty-four hours for seven full days. This means that I was connected to the IV pole and the chemo for a day. I was already attached for the antibiotics that I've been on for the sinus infection, but now I won't be off of the IV for a while. It is tougher when you have to unplug just to go to the bathroom or wait for the chemo treatment to be over so I can jump into the shower. I guess I will have to wait until tomorrow.

FRIDAY, JULY 5, 2013

We quickly decided that the best thing to do is to find a way to clearly communicate to everyone. Dave and my immediate family have been overwhelmed answering everyone's questions. We decided that the way to tell everyone what is going on is to create a blog-style form of communication that allows us to frequently update those who want to stay informed. This approach will work and will give Dave and my immediate family the ability to live life without constantly being asked the same questions over and over again. It will allow them to take care of themselves, too. This journey wasn't just hard for me; I know it was hard on them. We compiled a list of everyone we wanted to let know what was going on and sent out this email:

THE FIRST UPDATE

The Solomons' world just got turned upside down. On Friday, June 28, Mara went in to see her doctor for petechiae (a fancy term for broken blood vessels). They did some blood tests and, when she got them back Saturday morning, her white blood cells, red blood cells, and platelets were all very low. Mara was admitted to the hospital on Saturday, June 29. After two days of tests, CT scans, and a bone marrow biopsy/ aspiration, the preliminary results are pointing to Acute Myeloid Leukemia (AML). Mara had a central line put in on July 3 and began chemo on July 4. It is expected that she will be in the hospital for a month in isolation and hopefully achieve remission before she will be able to return home for some R&R. Then, over the next four months, she will go to the hospital for a week at a time every month to receive chemo treatments. As I'm sure you can understand, we are devastated by this sudden diagnosis and feel completely blindsided. We feel strongly that Mara will come through this with the great strength and determination that she has.

The purpose of this blog is two-fold. One is to provide all friends and family with updates of how Mara is battling this disease. The second purpose is to reach out to our wonderful community of friends and family for support in any way you can. We will be updating the calendar with opportunities to help to support our family with food, childcare, rides, etc. for those who are close by and able; and encouragement, prayers, kind thoughts, cards, or anything else spendable for those who are far away. Due to the fact that Mara is in isolation and at extremely high risk of infection, she is not allowed to have any fresh flowers, plants, fruits and vegetables, honey, raw nuts, etc. We have started a "we're all rooting for you" collage and would appreciate a picture of you to include to decorate her walls. In addition, Mara will be having many transfusions, as anyone with this type of disease needs, and although it is not possible to donate specifically to another person, donating to the blood reserves indirectly supports Mara.

We realize that this is likely to be a marathon rather than a sprint, and do so appreciate your friendship, love, and ongoing support through this difficult process.

Sending Love,
The Solomon Family

From this point forward, I began to make my day-to-day journal something that I sent to this great village of mine.

JULY 5, 2013
CHEMO DAY 2

I completed my first full 24 hours of chemo this morning, and I celebrated by getting to take a shower and wash my hair. Who knew that could be so exciting. With a catheter in my chest, I was under the impression that I was sponge bath bound for a while, but the nurses here were determined to let me enjoy a shower just to attempt to clean up. This whole shower thing is hard to do because I have to be extra careful not to get the central line wet. It takes at least 5 minutes to wrap me up to protect the line and keep it from getting wet.

Let me explain why I have to cover the central line and its lines in a cover. It consists of a 6" by 6" square piece of plastic with sticky tape around the sides. Imagine this, I am in my tank top (thank goodness I am not topless). I have to fold the two plastic lines that are dangling a few inches from a hole in my chest. Luckily these 2 lines have plastic caps on the end of them. To make them fit into the square plastic protector I need to fold them up. Once I get them folded up, I hold them in one hand carefully while I pick up the sticker with the other hand. I carefully put the sticker part under the 2 lines. Did I mention that the sticker part of the protector also needed to be unwrapped? Well add this into the job. I began the attachment using the stickered edges first pressing underneath then along each side and finally above my central lines. If you find this confusing reading this, you got through it much quicker than I did. Now, as exhausting as that was, it is totally worth it. I am so happy to finally be able to take a shower.

I'm stoked. I got to take a shower, but I spent the whole time trying not to get the wrapped-up part of my chest wet. That has me bending in all of these funny angles trying to wash my hair and get my body clean. Forget about the fact that I am still sore from getting the central line implanted into my chest. Thank goodness there isn't a video because I'm sure this looks ridiculous. Oh and then the towels that I have to wrap myself in. Think hotel towel size but smaller. Yes, can you imagine? I can barely wrap my hair up in it. I guess that won't be a problem when I have no hair, but for now it is a problem. How the heck am I expected to get my whole-body dry? Yes, good luck on that. I guess I should be happy that I am actually getting a shower. It has been 3 days since my last one. I know gross but a lot has gone on and apparently showering is not a priority to the hospital staff. I must have started to smell, so they realized it was about time I took one.

They started the second round of chemo at 11:45 a.m. this morning, and 9 hours later I'm feeling great, a little tired, but overall I've had a great day. I was able to walk around the hospital and use the pedal machine—you know one of those step things that you can pedal on while you are sitting down or at your desk? I could only use it for about 20 minutes because I got tired. Realistically I got bored, but it sounds better to say I am tired. It is ridiculous. It is not like I have anything else to do, so I must be bored. I'm trying to keep up my energy and strength while I can since I've been informed it will dwindle greatly over the next month.

When I was initially told that I was going to be in the hospital for a month, I was devastated about all of the milestones I'd be missing with the kids, like Eli's walking, talking, eating, and so much more. Well, today while Dave and the kids were here. We hung out in the open family waiting area. You are probably wondering why we wouldn't just get together in my hospital room. Remember how small the room was? It is so tough hanging out in my room on my own I can't imagine Eli in there with all of the lines and crawling on the dirty floor. There are so many nurses, doctors, nutrition people, cleaning people, trash people, and so many more all bringing their personal germs into the room. Not to mention all of the germs they get from the other rooms. It really is gross if you think about it. Hospitals are one of the most germ-infested places. Kind of odd if you think that you go there to get healthy and yet hospitals are so dirty.

That is why we have decided to hang out at the third floor family room. It is a nice open space with a couple couches, and it is often empty. We have found that the family room is the perfect place to hang out. Today we let the kids enjoy the open space to just be kids. Eli was enjoying couch surfing. You know, going from couch to couch helping her go around the room. Dave and I were talking and then out of nowhere, Eli let go of one of the couches and took her first steps. Yes, I got to witness Eli's first steps! Even though I was having to adapt to this new life away from my family here I was, here they were with me allowing me to witness her milestones. Yes, Eli's very first steps were being done in front of me. I will always remember this. It brought a sense of normalcy to this new out of control crazy life we were living. It allowed me a feeling of knowing that things are going to be okay, and I am not as removed from life as I really am and will be for a long time. It was amazing, and I'm so glad that I didn't have to miss out on that while here. After they went home, we began a new daily tradition of having dinner together over Skype, which was definitely a fun experience. I continue to be able to remain positive about where I am headed in this journey, and I am cautiously preparing myself for some of the next steps that I know will be challenging. Good night.

JULY 6, 2013
CHEMO DAY 3

I woke up at 3:30 a.m. this morning when the nurse took my vitals. Usually when they come in I either sleep through this process or go right back to sleep. Not this time. I wasn't able to go back to sleep. I just laid there and kept thinking about all that is going on right now. I cannot believe all that has happened in the last week. I am trying to find something good to focus my brain on, but I just can't. I really cannot believe all that I am going through right now.

One thing that I have to accept is that I have to live on the hospital schedule. Hence why I am being woken up at 3:30 a.m. The nurses have multiple shift changes throughout the day, and they have to do my vitals EVERY time the shift changes which is 3 times a day. Each time either a nurse comes in and takes my temperature, by putting a thermometer in my mouth for 30-60 seconds, then taking my blood pressure by wrapping a blood pressure cuff around my bicep. They Velcro it tightly around my arm and then the machine firmly squeezes my arm for a minute or so. Finally, they determine my oxygen levels by putting a clip on the tip of my middle or pointer finger to determine my overall oxygen levels. In addition, they ask me to breathe in and out while they put a stethoscope against my back and chest and ask me to take deep breaths in and out while they listen to my heart and lungs. This whole process takes 5-10 minutes. During the day this is no big deal. I enjoy chatting with the nurse catching up on things but in the middle of the night it is not the same. Some nurses are great. They respect that I am sleeping, and they quietly come into the room, dim the lights, and perform this shift change responsibility as quietly as they can. Other nurses have a different idea of how they should perform their duties. In the middle of the night this is very annoying, they must assume that since they are awake and working, I should be awake too. They come in, they turn on the lights, they say hello. Then they start talking to me while taking my vitals. In my mind I'm thinking: *Are you kidding me. I am trying to sleep here.* I'm not comfortable enough to be upfront with them. It is because of that loud nurse that I was wide awake and not able to go back to sleep.

It's hard to believe that it's been exactly a week since I first came into the hospital. So much has happened in 7 days. Not only have I started but I actually finished one of my chemo treatments today. I'm so excited to be done with the Idarubicin, and I will continue the Cytarabine through Thursday. My hemoglobin levels dropped today as we expected, so I had a blood transfusion in the afternoon. Normally a drop in hemoglobin would be considered dangerous and concerning, but I need to realize that the goal with the chemo is to decrease everything and essentially kill off the blood that my body is currently producing to get rid of the cancer. This is hard to wrap my head around. The great news is that with this infusion of blood I should have some additional energy, and I may be able to continue to feel good for another day.

The kids came by for a visit in the morning. It was fun to get to see them. I always look forward to their visits and am so fortunate that they fit a daily visit into their summer routine. I can't touch Eli at all because she is such a germ factory, but I can play peek a boo, blow kisses, and wave to her. I know it's hard for her to understand as she keeps reaching out for me when she's here. I have to say it is extremely hard for me too. These are my kids. We have such a physical bond and not being able to hold them both is so hard. All I want to do is hug Dave and the kids and I can't. Can you imagine not being able to hug your loved ones when you need them most? Not only are the doctors worried about my compromised immune system, but I am still in pain in my chest where I am still healing.

Alyssa is doing great but starting to push boundaries as she knows things are not going back to normal quickly. We've been talking to her a lot about what is happening, and how there are bad guys in my blood, and we are working to get rid of them so the good guys can take over again. She is asking questions, and we're really trying to be appropriately open with her, so she is as informed as she needs to be. She is and always has been a very mature four-year-old, which is great, but this is a lot for 30-year-olds to understand and accept. We want to keep her in the loop no more than she needs to be.

After what has become my version of a busy day, I'm hoping to call it a night early and get to sleep past 3:30 a.m. tomorrow morning.

We've been hearing everyone's love and support and know your compassion and love is helping us through this. It's so helpful to know that Dave and the kids are being taken care of while I'm here.

JULY 7, 2013
CHEMO DAY 4

I continued to receive the blood transfusion throughout the night last night. I was concerned this would make it hard for me to sleep since they were in the room at 1 a.m. and 3 a.m., fortunately I was able to sleep well. I woke up feeling really good. I had energy and was able to do my morning exercises, which includes riding a stationary bike (just the pedal part) and then after 7 a.m., I walk a few laps of the third floor of the hospital. It's nice because there's no one in the halls at that time, and I can just speed walk through with my IV pole attached to me. I'm determined to keep up my physical strength as long as I can. I have started to have some of my first chemo symptoms.

The skin on my hands is starting to peel. It's not painful yet, but it looks a bit creepy. Think Halloween costume peeling skin. On a positive note, my cultures all came back negative so after 6 days on IV antibiotics they have finally discontinued them. I don't have whatever infection they thought I might have had.

The kids did their daily visit, and Alyssa and I got a chance to color in her princess coloring book. Eli showed off a couple steps again, and she is looking so grown up.

I was moved to a bigger room this afternoon. The nurses have been telling me about this big room and they were keeping an eye on it for me. This morning my nurse said she thought it was going to free up today. Now unlike a hotel, the rooms aren't vacated by 11 a.m. However it is usually determined whether or not a patient is discharged after the doctors 10 a.m. rounds. I began packing up my belongings and eagerly awaited after my doctor completed his rounds. In the early afternoon I was informed that the room was open and had been cleaned. My nurse asked me to quickly finish packing up so I could get to the new room before they filled it with another patient. They didn't need to tell me twice; my suitcase was packed, and I rolled down the hallway to my new room. I had been told which room it was and that it was bigger, but I had never actually seen it, so I just had to take the nurses' words for it that it was a better room. Shoot, any room had to be better than my first one.

You aren't going to believe this. Let me describe it to you. As I opened the door, I quickly entered a washroom. It is a small closet-size rectangular room, maybe 4' wide by 10' long. It has a counter with a sink in it and cabinets above and below it. At the other end of the room is a tall wooden door with a window filling up the top half. I now know that this is a clean room to keep germs from staying out of or in the sterilized room. When I opened that door, my mouth dropped open and I was ecstatic. This room is amazing. Yes, I know I am still in a hospital, and I need to deal with all that is going on with being sick, but if I have to live in a hospital, this is life. Think penthouse of a hotel. This is the hospital penthouse. It is easily 4 times the size of my other room. The bed is placed centrally along the back wall. There are windows all along the other wall facing towards the trees, the lower hospital grounds and over past beyond the freeway. I know mentioning of the freeway doesn't sound pretty but it is great to see life beyond and also the gorgeous houses on the hills beyond. At the bottom part of the windows is a bench seat that ran the length of the window and allowed storage for the kids toys to stay when they aren't visiting. If that wasn't enough, no palatial suite would be complete without a huge bathroom. Not only does the bathroom have room for me to put my toiletries on my private sink and counter it also has a shower big enough to have a seat in it. Now I don't have any reason to use it but there is something nice about having a shower big enough for a seat. I don't think I've been this excited about a new room, but here I am very excited to get things up on the wall and get settled.

I so appreciate the expanding community and continued support that is helping me through this.

JULY 8, 2013
CHEMO DAY 5

I seem to be getting my morning routine underway, with the morning visits from nurses, doctors, etc., and taking care of my little exercise/ around the floor. I am able to entertain myself until about 8 a.m. each morning. I'm trying to find projects to keep me entertained. It's great that I feel good, I just need to figure out what I need to do to keep me busy. I'm considering picking up knitting again, but after my attempt to make Eli a baby blanket when I was pregnant. I'm wondering if knitting is not my calling. The blanket ended up being 3' by 20'. I'm not sure what happened but I need to try another hobby.

Dave and the kids came by, in the morning, and I was able to spend an hour and a bit coloring, playing, and doing the Macarena with Alyssa. It was just the two of us and it really was special. I had lower energy after they left and was starting to fall asleep when a nurse asked if she could get me anything. I let her know that I was fine, and then she said the magic words… "We have ice cream!" Next thing you know it's 11 a.m. and I'm eating chocolate ice cream. It was delicious. Who says you can't have dessert first?!

I was able to disconnect from chemo and those awful tubes today briefly so I could take an actual shower in my new, big shower. To make it even better, one of the nurses gave me a foot massage. The alone time, the foot massage, and having food delivered to me, allows me to momentarily think I'm at the spa and not the hospital.

JULY 9, 2013
CHEMO DAY 6

I had a bit of a tough night last night. That chest catheter that they put in last Wednesday, is still painful. I know I need this central line to deliver all of my meds, chemo, and blood more easily. It really is a good thing, but it is hurting me now. They say it's just scaring over, so I slept with an ice pack on my shoulder which was uncomfortable.

Today was pretty chill overall, Dave was able to come hang out for a few hours without the kids. It was nice to have a date day with him. I am excited to have completed day 5 of chemo and am well into day 6. Only one more day!

The genetic testing came back and showed that there were no genetic abnormalities. I'm not sure what that means overall. I like that it means it is not a scary type of AML, just the regular AML. I'm not sure if that is comforting or not but I will take it as good news. The one thing I like about that is that this is not something that I could be passing on to my kids. PHEW. These results also help with the overall prognosis, which means I will not be needing a bone marrow transplant. This is great news!

I've learned that the internet is intermittent during the day, which leaves me with plenty of time to watch movies and rest during the day. The kids came by in the evening to have dinner with me. Alyssa got to wear her new child-size masks that Dave had gotten for her, and Eli seemed to be in a pretty good mood. I am truly stretching to find things to entertain the kids. One thing that we found today was that thanks to the setting sun we were able to do shadow puppets on the wall which the kids enjoyed.

I'm looking forward to celebrating tomorrow as I get hooked on my final day of chemo for this session.

JULY 10, 2013
FINAL DAY OF CHEMO!

I was able to sleep in this morning and enjoy breakfast with the kids over Skype. This has turned out to be an easier time for us to Skype, so we can talk about what the day has in store for us all. Dr. S came in and discussed that they were not able to determine a subtype for my AML which he didn't seem to think was a big deal.

I was excited to learn that I can go outside again. This will be the first time that I've been outside in over a week. I still have to stay on the third floor, but there is a nice outdoor courtyard that I'm allowed to go out to. When the kids came, we were able to enjoy the courtyard and blow bubbles.

I was visited by the acupuncturist, and I hope to have the treatments along with the Jin Shin Jytsu. Like I said before, these are alternative medicine treatments I've been doing to help keep my energy up and reduce my side effects to the chemo. They seem to be helping. I guess I could put it this way. They are not not working.

Today they hooked me up to my last 24-hour dose of chemo and checked off day 7 on my calendar. It's exciting to be finishing things up with chemo for the time being. Dr. S said that now we will just wait until next Thursday when we do another bone marrow aspiration to get an idea of how effective the chemo has been. They have two goals at the moment. The first goal is to have my blood numbers drop and the second goal is for the aspiration to be clear of any leukemic cells.

The kids and Dave came by in the late afternoon, and Alyssa and Eli got to play doctor while the nurses took my vitals. Alyssa practiced flushing out my line. When Alyssa listened to my lungs, she told me I needed to stop breathing for a few minutes so she could hear what's going on. Thank goodness that's not part of the regular vitals protocol! I'm hoping to call it a night early and look forward to being detached from this central line tomorrow. The oncologist said that I could be completely detached from any wires for 24, 48, 72 hours or more as long as I don't get an infection and need antibiotics. Fingers crossed for some freedom! I'd love to walk without being attached to the pole. I'm clearly feeling everyone's support and love, and it's helping me continue to fight through.

JULY 10, 2013
THE HOME PERSPECTIVE

As Mara updates us on her amazing progress and fortitude, I thought it would be interesting to share the home perspective for Dave, Alyssa, Eli, and Brady (the dog). To say it has been an adjustment would be an understatement. Life at home has totally changed for all of us without Mara's presence here. She really is the glue that keeps things together for us.

Eli, of course, does not fully understand what is going on. When we visit Mara, she is always trying to reach out to her and wanting Mara to hold her. Alyssa has had a much more difficult time with this entire ordeal. She has been acting out a lot more (to be expected) and is needing a lot more attention.

Tuesday night was particularly challenging with Alyssa testing my patience. When I asked her why she was doing this, she said she missed her mommy and wanted her to come home. It broke my heart, and I explained we all just need to help each other out and get through this together as a family.

Dave (me) is trying to keep things at home as "normal" as possible. I am trying to make each day special for the kids and to keep us busy with fun activities and playdates. I enrolled both kids in swim lessons. Alyssa continues not to like putting her head under water, while Eli seems to enjoy the water more. In addition, Alyssa will be doing a musical day camp next week. It is *Tangled* (Rapunzel), which is her favorite right now. To make all of this happen, we decided to hire a part time nanny to help with the kids. This also allows Dave (me) to spend more time at the hospital with Mara. It is working out great so far, and we plan to continue for the next month.

Lastly, I wanted to personally thank everyone for all their support. From the meals, dog walks, visits, cards, emails, thoughts, and prayers, etc., the response has been more than I ever could have asked for. It is a great reminder of the strong network of family and friends we have all around us. Words can truly not express our deep-felt gratitude. We want our Mara back and we can't wait for the day that she is able to walk out of the hospital with us. We would not be able to achieve that goal without all of you.

JULY 11, 2013
ROUND 1 OF CHEMO COMPLETE!

BACK TO MARA'S PERSPECTIVE

Today is the day that I've been looking forward to since my diagnosis on July 2. I have geared up all of my energy to make sure that I can get through the 7 days of chemo. I realize this is just the beginning, but how the leukemia reacts to this chemo will determine how we move forward.

I was in a celebratory mood at 1:30 p.m. when they disconnected me from my chemo, and I was able to walk around without being attached to the IV pole. I realize this is the first time in 13 days I've been disconnected from the IV pole for more than a few minutes. This affords me the ability to walk around the room, the halls, and lay in bed without dragging along a separate set of wheels.

I spoke with my doctor about the waiting game ahead of me, and I got a dose of reality from the advanced practice nurse at the Oncology Clinic. She said she will be my new best friend for the next 5... yes 5... years. I realize that is just for overall monitoring ideally after a prompt remission, but it was still a bit of a reality check. Apparently 5 years is the magic amount of time that you need to be in remission for before you are considered cancer free. Now how they came up with 5 years I am not sure, but I will take it, Since I'm only 2 weeks into this horrible new life, 5 years sounds like an eternity. At least it gives me something to look forward to.

I'm definitely feeling fatigued throughout the day, but I seem to pick up my energy in the evening and am trying to keep up a routine to keep me motivated. Today, I was faced with the reality that we would not be doing our weeklong trip to Maine in August. Canceling those plane tickets was tough emotionally as we'd been looking forward to the trip since January. I also had to cancel our Hawaii trip that we had planned for Thanksgiving. That was also tough to do. Canceling these trips is making this become a reality. I think that in many ways I have put it in my mind that we can fix this. I keep forgetting how much it is affecting not just me but my immediate and extended family. Everyone is adapting their lives. Making us have to change our plans is showing me what a big deal it really is. To help me not go down a rabbit hole, I keep telling myself that we can replan both trips for next year when I will be less immunosuppressed and helps me be better accept all of these cancellations.

Dave was able to spend a good deal of time with me today, which was great, I got to go outside, and my mom brought the kids by in the afternoon. Alyssa diligently did my vitals again. I let her know that usually the doctors ask me to breathe when they listen to my lungs. Her response was, "Well, I'm not that kind of doctor. You can't breathe while I'm listening to your lungs." Fortunately, she hasn't figured out that I breathe the whole time anyway (don't tell her though).

JULY 12, 2013
THE WAITING GAME

Last night I had a dream. I escaped the hospital to go to a musical by myself, and I was rushing back through San Francisco to try to get back to the hospital before they noticed I was gone. That is the first dream I've had since I've been here. I guess this means I am officially able to sleep. What do you think this means?

Today marks 2 weeks since I went to the doctor to get my blood drawn. It's amazing how much our life has changed in 2 weeks. I mean seriously, 2 weeks ago I was planning for the Fourth of July and now I'm stuck in this hospital just hoping that I can get home.

My blood work today showed that my platelets were very low, so I received a platelet transfusion mid-morning, which meant I was attached to the pole again. Even though it was only for an hour, I'm so annoyed that I am connected to it again. I also feel so much better after a platelet transfusion. I seemed to have much more energy after it was complete.

The kids came for a quick visit before they headed out to Fairyland. Fairyland is a fun local kids park with story book settings, small friendly animals, and puppet shows. It is perfect for my kids ages. It is funny, it has been around forever. I went there as a kid, and it hasn't really changed. My kids seem to like it, and it is a great place for them to enjoy doing something other than hanging out with me in the hospital. Dave and my family are doing a great job making sure the kids are still able to enjoy being kids while still holding us together. I have to say this is so tough for me. I wish I could be out enjoying these fun experiences with them.

Before they headed out to Fairyland, the kids, Dave, and I got to enjoy the third floor courtyard where Alyssa picked flowers out there. If we go out there every day; there will be no more flowers by the time I leave.

I had a very positive meeting with my oncologist today. The original plan was to do another bone marrow aspiration/biopsy next Wednesday or Thursday. He said that he liked how my numbers were trending, and since the outcome of the bone marrow test wouldn't change my treatment regimen, he thought it was best to wait until Day 28 to do the biopsy/aspiration. This will prolong any update we receive about how the leukemia is responding to the chemo, but I'd prefer to wait until the 28th day anyway.

The other exciting thing about this news is that the day 28 bone marrow biopsy/ aspiration is an outpatient procedure. That means I will be out of the hospital by then, giving me a potential date of July 31 that I could be out of the hospital and home for a few days of R&R before starting my next in-patient chemo treatment! I'm so excited to not only know that I could go home but also to have dates to put on the calendar. It is so helpful to have actual dates to look forward to.

Although I've certainly been feeling a bit lethargic, today is one of the first days that I didn't really need a nap. My doctor wants me to exercise more (I really have no excuse to not exercise, I have all the time in the world) so I can keep up my strength. I may actually pull out one of my workout videos that I've been trying to use for almost a year but have never opened.

JULY 13, 2013
DAY 13

I didn't sleep great last night, which is a bit disappointing, but I was up and ready for the day at 6:30 a.m. I find that at night when I'm tired, everything seems to be uncomfortable. Usually that's when the nausea kicks in, or I get a headache. Last night I was waiting for my last antibiotic of the night around 10 p.m. and had to call my nurse to ask for every other medication I could take just because I wasn't comfortable. Fortunately, the anti-nausea medicine kicks in immediately and usually makes it so I can fall asleep right away.

This morning my only discomfort is something that feels kind of like a canker sore at the base of my tongue. It is amazing how much you use your tongue to talk and eat. Tylenol seems to make the discomfort tolerable, and they have a "magic mouthwash" that is made up of Mylanta and lidocaine and numbs my whole mouth to make my mouth comfortable at bedtime. As I type this my mouth is numb! I share this not only because it is what I am using but also because this magic mouthwash truly is magic. I swear this is so helpful if you are having difficulty with anything from talking to eating and even swallowing. I'm so glad they told me about it.

Dave brought the kids by this morning, and Eli took a few more steps to me today. It's so cute, and she's so proud of herself when she takes a few steps. We went back to the room and Alyssa did a paint by number with me and offered to put lotion on my feet. Of course I wasn't going to turn down a foot massage, but when it came down to it, she made my dad massage my feet. She just wanted to get the lotion. I guess she just wanted to tease me. I enjoyed the rest of the day and took it pretty easy.

I'm loving all of the cards, emails, and pictures. I am taping them up to my walls as soon as they arrive. One of these days I'll have to take a picture of my room, so everyone can see how they are a part of my recovery.

JULY 14, 2013
SUNDAY FUNDAY

The big drama of the day is my darn tongue. The on-call oncologist was concerned that I might have an abscess in my tongue (this would not be good). He called in an ENT, and fortunately the ENT was able to see that it is in fact a sore that is hidden on the base of my tongue. The good news is that it is nothing serious like cancer (few). The bad news is that it hurts like no other. Think of the pain of a canker sore but bigger at the base of your tongue. Can you relate? Well, it is driving me nuts and although I will power through it. It still hurts really bad and will probably last a few days. Since I am so immunosuppressed, I just have to wait it through. In the meantime, it affects everything I do with my mouth. Can you imagine me not talking? Fortunately, the doctor was able to figure that out before he had to do a CT scan or a scope down my nose. Now, not only do I get to use the magic mouthwash when I want, but I have topical lidocaine that I keep putting directly on to my tongue. I was afraid I would have to start eating all of my meals pureed, but with a little Tylenol and a little numbing, I can still eat my meals normally.

My blood numbers are looking good. I'm still neutropenic, but my numbers seem to be slowly recovering on their own. The more they come up, the better my immune system becomes and the better chance for me to go home by the end of the month.

The kids came by, and for the first time I spoke with Alyssa about how I am going to lose my hair. My doctor said that I should expect to lose it by day 10, and today is day 11, so my follicles have held strong for another day. I explained to Alyssa that I was going to get a really short haircut and shave my head like Daddy's. Oh, did I mention Dave is bald? She said, "So you'll be bald? That's going to look hilarious!" I told her we could go wig shopping when I'm out of the hospital, but she felt that wasn't necessary because we already have a wig at home that looks like Ms. Hannigan, and I could just wear that one. I'm not sure if I should take it as a compliment that she'd like me to look like Ms. Hannigan, but we'll go with that. At least she didn't recommend the Napoleon Dynamite wig!

JULY 15, 2013
ANOTHER DAY DRAMA FREE

I'm calling it a night early and didn't get a chance to write my update, so I'll write it tomorrow. I just didn't want people to worry if there wasn't an update. All is going well, and things are continuing to go in the right direction. I'll write more tomorrow morning.

JULY 16, 2013
QUICK JULY 15 NOTE

I didn't update yesterday because I was too tired, and everything was going well. I consider that a good thing. No news is good news, right? Now on to today!

This morning when I did FaceTime with Alyssa, the first thing she said to me was, "Hey, I thought you said you were going to shave your head. Why's your hair still there?" This is one of the most wonderful things about children and about Alyssa. She just puts it all in a new light and helps me not stress over the small stuff.

My tongue is still bugging me. Okay, it isn't just bugging me, it really hurts and prevents me from doing basic things without being in pain. At the same time, things overall are going really well. I started taking Tylenol with codeine and it makes it much easier for me to eat, talk, and feel pretty good overall. In general, I don't like to take pain medication, so this is unusual for me. At the same time, if I need to take these meds to be able to function I will.

As always, everyone's thoughts, prayers, and warm wishes are being felt, and clearly working to help me feel as good as possible throughout this chemo.

JULY 16, 2013
18 DAYS IN AND FEELING GREAT

I woke up this morning to some wonderful news! I have a new niece. She was born early this morning to Dave's brother and his wife. It's so wonderful to have something fun to celebrate amidst all of this craziness.

The rest of my day was certainly not that exciting but stayed looking good. The petechiae (fancy term for broken blood vessels) that I originally had when I was admitted to the hospital (it had since gone away) has come back and is worse than it was before. This led my doctor to order another platelet transfusion. Even though my platelets were at 12K, and they prefer not to transfuse until I get below 10K, he felt that it was necessary to get more platelets. My hemoglobin was also at 8 today, and my threshold for transfusion is <8, so they took my blood today to match me for a transfusion.

On that note, I've heard that some people have been able to donate blood to their local blood banks. This is fantastic, and I definitely appreciate you adding to the blood bank since I'm depleting their stock. Each transfusion is 2 bags worth. The more blood in the blood banks, the more people's lives you are saving.

I have had great nurses across the board, but there are 2 that I've taken a real liking to. One of them completely spoiled me and bought me a great comfortable throw for my bed. It's fantastic and so cuddly. I look forward to having it keep me warm at night instead of these sterile crispy hospital linens. It is great that with this blanket, the pillowcases from home and all of the cards around the walls this feels less sterile and more homely. The sad part is that it reminds me that I will be here a long time. I have to accept that I might as well just get comfortable since I will be here a while.

Fortunately, my mouth discomfort is much better today. I understand that mouth sores are a big part of being on chemo and seem to be the major side effect that I am experiencing. I'm more comfortable today and was able to go back to Tylenol as my main pain management medication. I also haven't made a big enough deal about being detached from the IV pole for 5 days now. WAHOO!

I topped the day off with an evening visit from the kids. It was short but enjoyable. Eli continues to take her couple steps here and there, and it's so rewarding that every time feels like it's her first steps (I think she's taking her time so I can keep enjoying the first steps over and over again). Alyssa helped me open more cards, and although she didn't have any zingers tonight, she was fun as always to hang out and color with.

JULY 17, 2013
ANOTHER DAY, ANOTHER TRANSFUSION

This morning my hemoglobin was down to 7.5, and if it's below 8 then they will give me a blood transfusion. They prepped me and were able to start the transfusion early, so I was attached to the pole again until 2 p.m. today. I definitely felt like I had less energy today then I've had the last couple days.

When the kids came by in the morning, I let Alyssa check out a new app on my iPad that she thought was pretty funny. The app was a cat that you could make do different activities. It would brush its teeth, and you helped it move the toothbrush up and down. Now if only I could get my kids to brush their teeth like the cat, that would be fantastic. As I write this it doesn't sound very fun but believe me it was hilarious. She liked it so much that she wanted to FaceTime with me in the evening, only because she thought she could play the game over FaceTime. I think she was a bit disappointed to learn she could only talk to me over FaceTime and not play the game at the same time.

I remained pretty lethargic for most of the day, which is unusual for me. They weighed me, and I'd lost 6 pounds since last week. Normally this would be a miracle in a good way. I've always been overweight and have worked hard throughout my life to lose weight. In this situation, it made me realize I have to bump up my eating. With my mouth hurting, I'm not able to eat as much as I should, and they would like me to. Fortunately, Dave brought the Magic Bullet (a small blender that I can put anything in) in to my room so we could blend up my food. I was then able to drink my soup and have a milkshake too. If I keep this up, I should be gaining that weight back really quickly. The nutritionist changed my diet to pureed only to help me increase what I could eat. Although I know this will mean I can eat more, it certainly doesn't make hospital food look any more appetizing. I remember a few days ago when I was happy that I didn't need to eat pureed food. Well now all of my food looks the same and they all need to be eaten with a straw. DISGUSTING. I hope this isn't for very long.

I have reached an all-new low today and watched *Honey Boo Boo*. I cannot believe I can't find anything better to do. I welcome any TV recommendations or ideas of other things I can do. My goodness I hope I have more energy and higher counts tomorrow so I can do more than just watch that show.

JULY 18, 2013
THE WAITING GAME CONTINUES

I woke up this morning feeling great! I had enough energy to… wait for it… turn on a workout video and actually do it! Yes, I was as surprised as everyone else is. I've been carrying this DVD in my computer bag for 9 months with the intention of doing the exercises at work and have never actually played the DVD until today. It was a good workout (only 20 minutes, and I took it easy). I turned on the video and stood in front of the screen. I stretched from the left to the right. I lifted my legs from side to side. I did jumping jacks, jumped up and down. I do many things I could do without having to touch the ground. Remember how dirty the hospital floors are? This was the first time that I actually felt my heart rate up since I've been here.

I was done with my exercise pretty early, so I could jump into my normal morning routine at 7 a.m. It started with my favorite, Face-Time with Dave and the kids. It's always fun to see them at their breakfast time, and we get to talk about what fun we all have in store for the day.

They have been coming over at 9 a.m. each morning which has been fun. They both love the app I was telling you about. Today the cat would repeat everything we said and did. Including things like funny things we would say. We would even brush its teeth, take a shower, and dry its hair. Eli likes to just pet the cat, and Alyssa likes to torture it. What does this say about my kids and their personalities?

My doctor adjusted my platelet transfusion numbers again. I used to get new platelets if I dropped below 10, then below 15, and now it has been adjusted to below 20. Today I'm at 26, so it's pretty likely I'll get more platelets tomorrow. My mouth continues to be the only part of me that is uncomfortable. Even though it is pretty uncomfortable, I feel very lucky that this is the only pain I'm experiencing, and it can be reduced greatly by medication. The doctor said it should continue or get worse over the next 10 days. I have to appreciate all that I am dealing with. I hear stories about different people's experiences, and I have to just take a minute to realize how lucky I am. I will have to stop complaining.

I also finished both my book and my first knitted headband last night. I did think that I'd give an easy knitting project a try and thought it would come in handy when the weather gets cooler. It was cool to have actually made something that I might actually use. I initially thought I would knit a hat. Isn't that what every basic knitter makes? Well apparently, I am not your average knitter. I made a very basic brown super small headband. Maybe it would fit an infant. With that, I am pleased I completed it. I hope it fits someone's small head. I may not be a professional knitter, but at least I gave it a shot and completed something, right?

I took it pretty easy today and laid low for most of the afternoon. I enjoyed a nice nap and a wonderful evening. I feel like I've finally figured out a successful nighttime routine that helps me stay as comfortable as possible while I sleep. I hope it continues to work. Everyone's cards, emails, etc. really keep me entertained. Don't ever feel you are bugging me with an email and an update on what is happening with you and your family this summer. I love living vicariously through you.

Also, for local people, we are looking for a nanny/babysitter who can watch the kids during the days starting in mid-August when Dave goes back to work. It would have to be someone who could come to our house every day and would be able to be flexible. Ideally, we'd like to have someone who we know, or one of our friends knows. If you know anyone who might be interested, please send me an email. Thanks!

JULY 19, 2013
8 DAYS DETACHED FROM THE IV

I woke up pretty energetic again this morning. First thing in the morning I got my blood work back and my platelets were low again. That is what we had expected, so I had a platelet transfusion. Up until now every transfusion I get raises my numbers, and then they come plummeting down pretty quickly. In the next couple days, we should see my numbers pick up with each transfusion and stay up. I'm so excited to see that my white blood cells are the highest they've been since I've been here. They are up to 1,800. The doctors say that once they are at 3,000 or higher I should be able to go home.

Playing the numbers game has been so strange. Initially my numbers were very low. That is how we knew there was a problem, that I had leukemia. That is why we started chemo to kill off the bad cancer. The goal then was to get me down to 0 or the fancy name I now know called "nadir." The reason you want 0 is because you want the bone marrow to no longer be producing leukemic blood. While achieving the lowest number of 0, we also wanted to make sure I had enough healthy red blood cells and platelets to keep me alive. This is why I continue to have blood and platelet transfusions from healthy donors. Are you following this? I ask because I know I am not sure I am. Once I hit nadir then the goal is for my blood marrow to be producing new blood cells that are cancer free. Ideally those healthy blood cells would be cancer free and now we are hoping the numbers would be higher and higher with cancer free blood. That is why we are cheering on an increase in the numbers every day when the blood is drawn. This will take time and should be worth the wait.

After labs, I was excited for the kids to do their usual daily visit. First, they came in the morning, then they left for Alyssa to perform in her summer camp performance of *Tangled*. I was bummed that I couldn't go to the performance, but Dave took a video of it, and I got to watch it with Alyssa afterwards. The musical was *Tangled*, and she had the role of the second chameleon, Leonardo. She did a great job. One of her strengths is being able to project her lines very clearly. She loves to perform and had a great time this week at the camp.

I took it easy in the afternoon and evening. I've been craving a smoothie lately, but of course due to smoothies having fresh fruit in them, I can't eat it. However, I figured out that with my small blender in my room I could make a smoothie with the yogurt and the canned fruit that they serve me during my meals. It wasn't the best smoothie ever, but certainly tasted good, and was much better than the pureed pot roast they served for dinner.

I don't know if I have told you about my fridge. The hospital room doesn't come with a fridge or blender, but since I am here for a long time, I am really trying to make this as homey as I can. I had a small fridge at home that I wasn't using for anything, so we figured what better way to use it then to bring it into my hospital room. I have been using it to keep all of the extra food that people have brought me or that I haven't eaten during my meals. I hate wasting food, and here I can store them for later and don't have to throw them away.

JULY 20, 2013
THE DAY I'VE DREADED

I have dreaded this day ever since my initial diagnosis. On July 2 when my doctor told me I had leukemia, my first question before I asked anything about the disease was "Will I lose my hair?" The answer was yes.

Even though everyone says it's just hair, and it will grow back, being faced with losing all of my hair was very difficult for me. We let ourselves be defined by our hair. If we have a great hair day, we have a great day; a bad hair day can put a damper on the whole day. I've decided that I'll no longer be able to define myself by my hair but instead have to be defined by my winning personality!

I knew we had to shave my head today because, last night when I ran my fingers through my hair, I noticed that 20+ hairs were coming out at a time. The nurses let me know that the hair will start coming out in chunks, and it can be difficult to see it happen. I tied my hair back in a ponytail and let Dave know that today would be the day that we shave my head.

One of the reasons I was so concerned about losing my hair was because throughout the last 3 weeks I've felt very good, all things considered. I don't think I look sick, but once my hair is gone, then I will look sick. In the past week, I've really changed my opinion on this. Since everything about this diagnosis is out of my control, I had to be in charge of when and how this was going to happen. Instead of looking sick, I think this no hair look really represents what I've been through and risen above. When Dave came in with the kids today, he had the honor of shaving my head (I've been shaving his for 10 years, so it's about time he got to be my hairdresser). The nurses said he should keep a guard on the shaver (so I don't accidentally get cut), so it is a #1 buzz cut. We went into my bathroom and as he pulled out the electric razor, I took one last look at my slowly thinning hair and told him to go for it. He started at the front middle of my forehead and slowly went throughout my head. The clumps of hair fell down the front and sides of my head and onto the floor. It wasn't as emotional as I thought it would be. I made sure that he didn't leave any clumps, and I made sure he went to all of the areas so it didn't look patchy. To help me feel comfortable, I did his hair too. Look at us. We were now twinning. I have to say I like how I look a lot more than I ever thought I would. I feel kind of like GI Jane.

I had let Alyssa know that today was the day I was going to cut my hair so that she wouldn't be surprised when she saw me. In typical Alyssa fashion, when I first stepped out with my new shaved head, she told me that I looked funny, and then asked if she could shave her head too! Eli didn't recognize me for a minute, but after I kept talking to her and let her touch my hair, she seemed to be happy.

Alyssa has a new fun project now when she visits me. You see, being neutropenic I've not been allowed to shave my legs for 3 weeks now. Alyssa has been letting me know that my legs are REALLY hairy. Well today I let her know an interesting fact about chemo. Not only does it make the hair on my head fall out, but it also affects my leg hair. She thinks it's so cool that she can just pull on my leg hairs and they come right out. I see hours of entertainment ahead of us!

JULY 21, 2013
THREE WEEKS DOWN

Today was a great day. I was planning on having to have a blood transfusion today because my hemoglobin was at 8.8 yesterday. Fortunately, my hemoglobin was at 9 today so I didn't have to think about a transfusion which was nice. Remember how the goal is to have my numbers trending up? I am so happy that they are!

I had a great time FaceTiming with the kids at breakfast and had a wonderful visit with them when they came by later. Eli has been doing very well throughout this whole ordeal, but it is clear that she is missing having both Dave and me at home. She knows I'm sick, and she is trying to get a handle on the whole situation.

Alyssa and I read two books about a mom who has cancer. One was written from the mom's perspective and the other from the kids' perspective. Fortunately, I had read these books earlier in the week, so I was able to read them with Alyssa without balling throughout it. These books really helped open up the conversation with Alyssa to speak openly about everything we are dealing with. We could both talk about how cancer is scary and can make us all sad. They shared how I'll be back home soon, and we can play games, cuddle, and spend lots of time together. For a four-year-old, Alyssa does a very good job of expressing emotion. We are going to do more mommy and Alyssa time while I'm in the hospital, and tons more once I get home.

The rest of the day continued to be really relaxing. I was able to hang out with Dave for 4 hours today. I know I relaxed a lot lately, but it's really nice to have company to relax with, and I know for Dave it's great for him to be able to just put his feet up for a few hours. I'm excited to see that ideally I only have 9 more days here. I am doing everything within my control to make that happen. The main thing I need to do is increase my blood counts across the board. I've been pretty steady the last day or two and am looking forward to the uptick. We put up a couple more pictures on the walls. I will keep adding photos so I can see how everyone is doing in picture format.

JULY 22, 2013
THE HOME STRETCH

This morning Dr. S gave me some potentially great news. He told me not to get my hopes up, but that if my numbers increase and I continue to be doing well I could possibly go home on Friday, July 26. WAHOO! YIPPEE! YEAH! I'm SO EXCITED!

I have to admit I've been quite excited about this all day and hope that I continue to do as well as I have been so I can go home on Friday. And, if for some reason that can't happen, the original plan to go home on July 30 is only 4 days later.

I had a great time FaceTiming with the kids this morning. Eli grunted at me as usual, and Alyssa told me in extremely dramatic fashion how she injured her quad and wasn't sure if she would be able to walk. She was so matter of fact about it. I had her bring an ace wrap with her when she came to visit, and low and behold, an ace wrap and a little Tylenol solved her pain for the whole day. My mom did remind me tonight of all of my "injuries" I had as a kid. I always had an ace wrap, a sling, a crutch, or something to help relieve/display my different ailments.

In the evening, I went for a walk and met another woman around my age with 2 young kids who is toward the end of her treatments.

She's been going through this for at least 6 months. There was something very reassuring about meeting this woman. I really appreciated knowing that I was not alone. Knowing that she was successful and able to have this terrible disease and be okay. Her family was okay and all she had to do was come into the hospital every couple weeks. This gave me great hope. Up until now I've not met any other patients, and I've not really been ready to speak with others who had or are experiencing leukemia. Up until now I've not really looked into the resources available to me once I get out of the hospital just because I didn't want to get my hopes up. I think I am ready to look into what is available for me.

I heard about a great cancer support community that is conveniently very close to where we live. Now that my departure date is getting closer, I'm ready to check these things out for myself and my family.

I am just finishing up today's update, and you won't believe this. The fire alarm is going off as I write this, oh crap, what should I do? I am sitting in my bed, in my double doored room, and the fire alarm is going off. I feel stuck. Should I run to the door? Should I run out to the hallway? I hear the hallway doors shutting. I assume this is to prevent fire from spreading, but if the fire is in my area, that could keep me stuck with the fire. I have to say, instead of feeling safe, I feel completely helpless. Should I call the nurses station? No one is coming to save me, so I guess I'm okay, but it really is nerve-racking.

This has happened previously, and the announcement said first floor. Okay no big deal. I assume it is the kitchen, but the announcement this time is saying third floor central. Well, I reside on the third floor central. I stood looking out my window to see if anyone seemed shocked or was trying to get me out, and I finally put on a mask and went to the nurses' station where they were just sitting there going about their business while the alarm went off. They weren't sure if it was a drill, but they thought it was. It made me realize, when you go on a cruise you have to go through the whole emergency drills. Shoot, even my office building makes us do fire drills. When I checked into the hospital, they never told me what to do when the fire alarm goes off. Apparently, I just keep doing what I'm doing and hope the alarm goes off (sounds like a real smart plan!). I guess if I don't do an update tomorrow, you will know what happened.

JULY 23, 2013
QUICK UPDATE

I had another good day. Dr. S came back and still feels that Friday is the day for me to leave even if my numbers don't pick up. He said I will have another blood transfusion before I go home just to make sure I go home with good high numbers. I also have 4 appointments set up for next week at the outpatient clinic. I had a platelet transfusion today that not only will pick up my platelet count, but also give me a nice boost of energy in the early afternoon. The kids switched it up and came in the evening which was fun. They were superstars and had a great time. I'm ready for bed but will write more tomorrow. Have a great night.

JULY 24, 2013
THE FIRST SET BACK

Today was one of the first setbacks I've experienced since I received my diagnosis. Last night when I was going to bed, I had a low-grade fever of 99.5 (I'm usually 97.3-98.3). When they checked it again at midnight, I was at 100, and at 4 a.m. I was at 101. Unfortunately, I knew exactly what this meant. It means that I probably have an infection of some sort, which means I can't go home on Friday. I was crushed, although I have some apprehension about going home just because I'll need to work out a routine and manage my own medications, pain, etc. and make sure I don't overdo it.

As the day went on and I talked to some of my awesome nurses I came to realize it's actually a good thing that this happened now. Obviously, I'd prefer to have not had any infection, but it would be devastating to get out of the hospital, only to get a fever at home and have to come right back to the hospital. At least I didn't have to move out of my "luxurious" room.

They took blood cultures at 4 a.m. and 5 a.m., and I should have preliminary results of what the infection is in 24 hours and more definitive results in 5 days. When Dr. S came in, he confirmed I will not be going home for at least 5 days and I'm back on the pole for most of the day as they give me 3 separate antibiotics via IV.

I didn't sleep well last night because I was hot and cold and just overall uncomfortable, so today I had very low energy. I had a later than usual FaceTime with the kids, which meant that they weren't at the table. Usually, Eli sits in her highchair and grunts/yells at me from there. Today they were in the family room, and Eli kept trying to hug me through FaceTime.

Not to brag, but my kids are REALLY cute. They visited me later in the afternoon, and we got to go to the courtyard and experience the heat outside. It was hotter than I liked outside, so I made the court-yard visit quick and we played for a minute then went back into the nicely air-conditioned hospital.

I had to have a chest X-ray in the afternoon. I thought that I was going to have to get into a wheelchair and be wheeled downstairs. However, it was a completely different experience. The X-ray tech-nician came directly to my room. They had me sit up in bed and placed a board behind my back and brought an x- ray camera in front of my chest. The whole process took less than 5 minutes. I know it is the little things, but this really was nice that they came to me. To help normalize all of these strange things I am going through, I talked to the technician to understand what he was doing. He was not interested in talking to me, so I stopped. What I under-stand though is that I needed this X-ray to make sure that my lungs are not cloudy, and the fever is not pneumonia or any issues with my lungs. That is all I know, and I guess we will find out more if they see anything with the results from the X-rays.

As the night went on, I got my bedtime temperature taken at 9:45 p.m. and it was back up to 101. We've got to get this fever down and let these antibiotics kill whatever infection is occurring right now.

With that I wish you a wonderful night, and thank you all for the overwhelming support, keeping my husband and kids fed, and the dog walked. It's been so nice for Dave to not have to worry about that on top of taking care of the kids on his own and taking care of me.

JULY 25, 2013
RIDING OUT THE FEVER

I had a pretty good night last night; this was great since I have an odd routine during the nights in the hospital. My routine consists of, going to sleep at 10, then I sleep for a few hours, get woken up for vitals, then decide to be wide awake and need to eat. At 1 a.m. I drink my little energy shake. Then I go back to bed. Is that normal? Who knows, but it has become my new normal.

Last night I was a bit more chatty than usual because it turns out my night nurse used to live in New Zealand. I love that because I have lived there too. We exchanged stories about how much fun we each had in NZ. That probably didn't help me fall right back to sleep. It totally threw off my usual night routine.

My blood count is improving slowly, the white blood cells were the highest they've been since before I got my first blood test. They are at 3.2. My hemoglobin continues to hover above 8 and is slowly increasing. Nothing massive, but it's looking good. The blood cultures that they drew yesterday have shown that I have a bacterial infection. They will continue to grow it over the weekend to get a better idea of what is going on.

I continue to only have discomfort in my mouth and face. My tongue is much more comfortable than it has been over the last 3 weeks. Even though the tongue is better, I now have half of my bottom lip extremely swollen. It looks a bit like Angelina Jolie's lip (if she only had half of her bottom lip really plump and cracked). Can you picture it now?

Dave and I decided not to have the kids come by to visit today. Eli seemed a bit fussy, and I didn't want to catch anything if she was sick and vice versa. This is the first day since my diagnosis that they haven't come and visited. Fortunately, we were able to FaceTime a few times today, which was nice and made up for not seeing them in person.

Unfortunately, my fever keeps coming back throughout the day. By 9 p.m. it was back up to 101 (it's usually at its highest at night). We're waiting to hear back from the on-call oncologist to see what to do. I'm already on every antibiotic under that sun, so they may be just waiting some of this out while trying to reduce the fever with Tylenol.

I've not been talking about it, but I've been continuing my exercising. Apparently, I got a bit overzealous with my squats because yesterday and today I've been so sore in my glutes, but I continue to push through the pain. The fact that I'd be sore from 15 squats that I may have held for 5 seconds each is pretty funny. I'll clearly have to step up my routine day after day. Oh, on another exciting note, I have a new neighbor who is a screamer. She doesn't seem to be in pain and doesn't seem to be overly happy; they just seem to be randomly screaming. Hopefully they sleep well or are able to be better medicated during the night. Better yet, I should be drugged up enough that it won't faze me.

JULY 26, 2013
ANOTHER DAY, ANOTHER FEVER

I had another great night's sleep last night. I guess the screamer either didn't scream or it didn't affect me. Even though the nurses were changing out my antibiotics throughout the night, I was able to basically sleep while they changed IVs. I slept so well that I was up for the day at 5:50 a.m. Thank goodness I was up early because if I hadn't woken up on my own, I would have been woken up at 5:59 a.m. by the fire alarm. Yes, another fire alarm! I've come to not let them freak me out.

My fever continued to present itself throughout the day with a high of 102.5. I'm on 3 IV antibiotics still and will be through the weekend and probably into next week. I cannot go home until I've been fever free for 24 hours. I'm sure I will also need to finish this course of antibiotics, but I am not sure how long this course will be.

The kids came by in the early afternoon. It was great even though Eli was fussy because she hadn't napped well. We got to walk around and hang out outside in the courtyard for a bit. Whenever Eli would get fussy, we would rely on the animal app that we had, and she was immediately distracted. Thank goodness for screens, I guess.

I had just finished knitting my second headband, when Alyssa decided she wanted to knit she took a knitting needle and wrapped the yarn around it until it was done. She was so proud that she could knit. Apparently wrapping the yarn around the needle was knitting. I didn't want to tell her that there was more to knitting than that because after roughly 2 minutes of wrapping the yarn around the needle she was done.

My GI Jane haircut is thinning as the days go on. I'm shedding like a dog and am curious how long it will take for all of my hair to fall out. I will continue to rock the thinning hair look until it becomes out of control, and then I'll need to come up with a new name for the look.

I'm really focusing on pain management and getting rid of this fever. Have a wonderful weekend!

JULY 27, 2013
TRANSFUSION DAY!

I'm writing tonight's update before I take my meds, so hopefully I can stay awake while writing it. It's bad when my updates are even putting me to sleep!

This morning, I woke up bright and early after another good night's sleep. I continued to have a low-grade fever throughout the night that has continued throughout the day. I've had 4 cultures done to determine what type of infection I have. Two cultures were done on Wednesday: one from my central line and one from my arm. One of those came back positive for a bacterial infection and the other one came back negative. Unfortunately, it seems they didn't know which culture was from my arm and which was from the central line, so they redid the cultures on Thursday. One of those has come back negative and we are waiting for the fourth. I learned that there's a chance that my fever isn't related to an infection at all and is just a chemo fever. They've been loading me up on every type of antibiotic; it would be nice to get to stop those. Normally I would be upset... even furious... but I think a part of me has just learned to accept things. They are what they are, and things will be what they will be. This should be my new motto.

Overall, I'm feeling pretty good. My hemoglobin was down to 7.7 today so I received a transfusion in the late afternoon. Even with low hemoglobin, I had a lot of energy today. As soon as I find out that my numbers are low enough that I need blood then they have to draw additional blood so they can cross-type my blood with the donor blood. The cross-typing can take a couple hours and then they have to get blood that's an exact match that they have to "clean" to make sure that there is no chance of rejection. The transfusion process takes a long time. I find it funny how donating a pint of blood can take as little as 5 minutes once you are hooked up. But the process of receiving blood takes hours. As soon as they determine that you require a blood transfusion, they take your blood to determine what type of match you need. Then they reach out to the blood bank. This can take between 30-90 minutes. I am sure it can be quicker, but since in my case it is not an emergency, they don't rush it. Then once they bring it into the room, hook it up. Two nurses have paperwork and match the blood in the bag to my blood type. I am very grateful that they take these extra steps. I take for granted how important it is that they are putting the correct type of blood into my body. I am A+ blood so I can only receive A+, A-, or universal blood donors O. After the two nurses have received the correct blood for me, they then hang the bag of blood onto the IV pole attach my line to the IV and it takes about an hour or two for the pint of blood to flow into my body. The process of donating and receiving platelets is the opposite. The time to donate platelets once hooked up is about 2 hours yet receiving them once matched etc. is about 5 minutes. Isn't that interesting?

I realize that I've been in the hospital for 4 full weeks now, and I really don't have much to show for it. I had thought that I would have read a few books, learned to knit new patterns, etc. I've now knitted 2 headbands, watched a few movies, finished 1 book and started another, and I think that is it. My biggest accomplishment occurred today. I organized my junk pile from home.

In our kitchen at home, we have this huge pile of mail and "important papers" that I haven't gotten around to filing. Yesterday my mom boxed it up and brought it over to me. Today I had the plea-sure of organizing it, and I'm embarrassed to say it looks like some of this mail had been sitting there for a whole year (oops!). Well, it is now organized, and the important stuff could be married down to one small file worth of stuff. It is so funny how I thought things were so important I had to hold on to it.

The kiddos came in the evening and were loud and boisterous as ever. Eli has learned to find the iPad as soon as she gets to the room. She also goes straight to the snack cabinet. She's getting closer and closer to walking as her confidence increases, but overall she is a much faster crawler. Alyssa was all about hanging all over Eli. I know that she sees the attention that Eli gets for taking steps and she wants the attention, so she hangs all over her. Towards the end of the visit, I sat her down to talk to her. I told her that she and Eli get to play together and wrestle all the time, but I only get to see her for a little bit each day and when she's visiting, I want her attention because I don't get to play with her all the time. We will see how that plays out tomorrow.

Speaking of tomorrow, tomorrow is my birthday, and although I had not planned to spend my 34th birthday in the hospital. With that change in plans, I will make sure I can make as big of a deal about it as I can. You see, my birth sign is Leo, and us Leos like to be the center of attention, especially on our birthdays. I am sure I will celebrate in the hospital as well as when I get home. I definitely know what my wish will be when I blow out the candles, and hope-fully I don't set off the fire alarm! Have a great Sunday!

JULY 28, 2013
HAPPY BIRTHDAY TO ME!

As I said yesterday, this is not how I thought I would be celebrating my 34th birthday. I had imagined bringing in my birthday morning with the kiddos in bed with Dave, all singing happy birthday, maybe a hot cup of coffee and a nice walk to the park. Oh, how I so badly wish I could be doing this now.

Instead, I had a rough night of sleep last night. All night, they were switching out the antibiotics and the final bag of blood for my blood transfusion throughout the night. I was still attached to the IV pole until 9 a.m. I guess that was my birthday treat. I was able to be detached from the IV pole. I did also get that birthday cup of coffee I so hoped for. By the time the coffee came to my room, it was luke-warm. At least I was in bed like I had imagined. That was what I wanted right?

The nurses had monitored me closely all night and throughout the day. My white blood cells continue to get higher day after day. My darn fever continued throughout most of the day until midafter-noon when I finally cooled down to 98.6 and have stayed around there since about 4 p.m. I have to be fever free for 24 hours before they will consider sending me home. We also received the 4th culture back which was negative, so apparently, I do not have an infection. We may never know what the fever was from. I am now very focused (some may say psychotically obsessed) on this bone marrow aspiration because the outcome of that really determines my next steps and how we tackle this disease.

Now onto the fun stuff. Today was a great day! I was overwhelmed with phone calls, emails, and Facebook messages wishing me a happy birthday. The nurses even got in on the birthday celebrations and both the day and evening shifts all came in singing Happy Birthday. It was really sweet. My parents brought some balloons that the kids thought were the coolest things ever, and Eli just kept playing with and trying to have all three balloons in her hands at once.

Alyssa was so cute as she kept wishing me happy birthday every time we talked: in the morning, when she visited, and in the evening. For the last call she said, "Happy Birthday! Can you believe it is still your birthday?" We had ice cream cake. This is my favorite cake, and I was able to enjoy every bite of it. I wasn't able to have candles lit up on it for fire protection. At least that is what they told me, but that didn't stop me. We put the candles on, and I made the most important wish I've ever made before I blew out the pretend flames. Now I am not supposed to tell you what my wish was, and I won't because I NEED this wish to come true.

JULY 29, 2013
28 DAY BONE MARROW ASPIRATION/BIOPSY

Today was a very tough day that reminds me of the importance of taking things one day at a time and to learn how to be accepting when things do not go the exact way I want them to. Turns out that my daily blood tests yesterday showed 1% blast/immature cells. This is bad news. The immature/blast cells could be an indicator that leukemia is still in my body, and I am not in remission as planned. I say could, because I am really hoping that this is a mistake. I hope they didn't see the blasts. The only real way to tell if the leukemia is still in my blood is to do a bone marrow biopsy/aspiration, so this afternoon I had the procedure done. This is not the birthday present I wanted.

I've been very anxious about what the bone marrow biopsy results will show. I'm happy that I don't have to wait until Thursday or next Monday (when the original biopsy appointments were scheduled) to get the test done. Dr. S did say that he has had other patients who presented with blast cells in the blood and the leukemia was in remission. Today there were no blast cells in my blood, but we need to be prepared for all possible outcomes.

Normally after the biopsy we are able to get preliminary results in 24 hours. Since my bone marrow has been obliterated by the chemo and is in the process of growing back, the aspiration showed very little bone marrow and most of that was blood. Since it didn't give them everything, they needed to make a clear diagnosis. That leads them to rely on the biopsy, which was a piece of my bone that will take 48-56 hours before we have information as to whether leukemia is still lingering in the bone marrow or has been obliterated and I am in remission.

This was obviously very difficult to deal with today. I continue to push back my goal date of when I get to go home. Tuesday the 30th was my original go home date. Since I was doing so well, I got my hopes up that I could go home on the 26th. Now I need to accept that things change. I am now aiming to go home on August 2. I will keep aiming for that. I am definitely ready to go home, even if it is only for a few days. If the bone marrow results are negative (there is no sign of leukemia) then I will be able to go home for a few days before I come back to the hospital for a short chemo consolidation treatment that will keep me in the hospital for 5 days. If the results are positive (I still have leukemia) I will hopefully get to go home for a few days, but I will have to return to the hospital for another month of treatment. That treatment will consist of the 2 chemos at the same time: one that is 3 days, for 15 minutes each day and the other that is 7 doses with each lasting 24 hours.

You are probably wondering why I am asking for and thinking about all of these different options and not just waiting for the results. The reason is this whole thing is a waiting game. Although all that I need to worry about is what they tell me to do, every result of these tests not only affects me, it affects my family and everyone involved in these. How is Dave going to go back to work, who is going to watch the kids? They can't go back to daycare; that is a germ factory.

While I had been thinking through all of these different scenarios, Dr. S came in to tell me the temporary results of my biopsy. Things were not looking good. Shortly after I received the bad news, Dave and the kids arrived. Alyssa took one look at me and asked, "Mommy, why are you crying?" How do you answer that? How do you tell your four-year-old daughter that her mother, who has been in the hospital for the last month, may be coming home for a week and then will have to go back to the hospital for a month? I tried to break it down as simply as I could. I told her that the bad guys that were in my blood are still there, and I might not get to go home as quickly as I wanted.

She hugged me tightly. I asked her if she wanted to color, and she asked, "Did you say cuddle?" Sure, enough we sat and read a book and cuddled for a bit until Eli was melting down enough that Dave had to take them home. I was lucky Dave got to come back after dropping the kids off at home, and he stayed with me for the whole day. I swear he stays here for the ginger ale and the good pizza conveniently located across the street, but I don't care. I love his company.

I know I've been asking for positive thoughts all along, and clearly, they have worked because regardless of the outcome of the bone marrow, I have been feeling great throughout this whole process. I attribute that to this incredible group of friends and family I have supporting me. With all of your prayers and positive thoughts, please wish with me for a NEGATIVE result from the bone marrow biopsy.

JULY 30, 2013
A GREAT DAY WHILE WE WAIT

I had a very good night of sleep and woke up this morning with great energy. I did my exercises as usual, and I was feeling really good. That is one of the bizarre things about this journey. Here I am with this horrific diagnosis, and yet I feel fantastic overall.

My mouth stuff has gotten a ton better over the last week, and I have taken myself off the pureed meals and actually can eat some of the normal foods like pasta, mashed potatoes and gravy, steamed vegetables, etc. Who knew I would be raving about hospital food, but normal hospital food is much better than pureed hospital food? Fortunately, ice cream is still included in the list of things that I am encouraged to eat, and I have some ready for me to gobble up.

Last night the kids spent the night at my parents' house. This is the first time that both kids have stayed there. This turned out to be a fun night for Grandma and Papa, and the kids had a blast too. This also meant that Dave got a night off, so he was able to not have to worry about the kids and take it easy. He even got to walk Brady (our dog) on his own without the kids with him.

This morning was like the good old days before I got sick. The only difference was that we were in the hospital and not at home. The kids came and joined me and Dave and my mom at my room at 9ish. The kids and I had fun. Eli kept working on her walking; she takes about 7 steps at a time and then she crawls straight to the snack cabinet and pulls out a bunch of snacks. I tried to teach Alyssa the "Cups" song and the pattern for tapping the cup while you sing. She got the beginning, but then was done with it. Eli was also very interested in the "Cups" song but just wanted to push the cup around. They will eventually get it.

The kids left to get on with their day, and I took a walk around the third floor. It was so fun; I knew many people throughout the halls, so I kept getting stopped seeing a different nurse or doctor and getting caught up. The cleaning crew wanted to show me how much they clean during the day. It was kind of fun, and clearly showed I've been here too long if I know people in every wing of the third floor.

When I returned to the room, I received a call from none other than the Red Cross asking me to make an appointment for my next blood donation. I once again find it ironic that I used to be a consistent blood donor. After explaining to her that I would no longer be an appropriate donor, she completed the call saying she would call me back in 2 years. I'm 100% positive that they would no longer be interested in my blood, but if she needed to, she could keep me on her list.

Another thing that made my day fantastic was that Dave was able to again spend much of the day with me. We were able to enjoy the nice weather outside and play Scrabble. Dave beat me by over 100 points, but only because he got 2 bingos! I firmly believe that I let him win! (As you may know I very rarely win Scrabble against Dave).

As the day went on, I had a weird discomfort in my Achilles tendon, up through the back of my knee. By bedtime it was excruciating; I couldn't even put weight on it. The on-call oncologist had me put my leg up and on ice. It is always so frustrating; I really had a fantastic day, felt I've made great headway, and then by the end of

the night, I'm back in the middle of a whole new ailment. I'm definitely keeping everyone guessing, and certainly confirming with
myself that it is a good thing that I didn't go home like I had originally thought I would. It would have been awful because I would
have had to come back into the hospital for each of these ailments.
The fever, this Achilles ailment, and who knows what else would
have happened if I went home. At least I get to stay in my comfy
penthouse suite at the hospital while we try to figure out what is
going on. This is also a distraction from waiting for the biopsy to get
back. Hopefully this Achilles injury is just a fluke and maybe I
twisted my ankle during my social walk around the floor, and it is
just swollen and sore from that. The long awaited for biopsy results
should be here tomorrow.

JULY 31, 2013
NOT THE DAY I HAD PLANNED ON

I spent the night with my foot raised on pillows and on an ice pack. I was not able to put weight on my right foot this morning. As the morning went on somehow, I was able to carefully walk with a limp, but at least I could gimp along, which is much better than being stuck in bed. They are thinking this could be either related to antibiotics that I am on or could be similar to the other odd pains I've had in my chin and back that were randomly extremely sore and swollen and then went away as quickly as they had arrived. Just another bump in the road and possible delay to me going home.

My oncologist paid me a visit around 9 a.m. with an update on my biopsy results. Unfortunately, the leukemia is still present, and we now need to explore our next course of treatment. In the very preliminary results, they found that there are 3% of blast cells in the blood. When I originally came in, I had 18% so the numbers are better, but what we needed for me to be in remission which would show 0% blasts. The pathologist will continue looking at the bone marrow from the biopsy, but it will take a few more days before they will be able to get an accurate count. If they see blasts in the preliminary biopsy that means that they are sure to see many more as they look at the marrow further.

If you are like me, you are probably wondering, well, what the &*%$#@ do we do now? I had originally thought that if I was not in remission, we would immediately start up the same course of treatment that I did this time to get the remaining leukemia out of my body. It turns out there are many options, and it will take up to a week to determine which treatment options might be best for me. The first and possibly most ideal next step would be a bone marrow transplant (BMT).

When I was first diagnosed, I thought that chemo was the route I would go, and bone marrow transplant required you to be in remission. I didn't do much research previously about a BMT because I have been convinced that chemo was going to put me into remission. With this news the best thing for me to do is to start digging into what a BMT is, where I can get it and what are my next steps. I am now researching how a BMT works and what I need to do.

What I have learned and understand so far is, there are 2 types of BMT. An autologous transplant and an allogeneic transplant. For the autologous transplant, they will give me chemo to get me back down to nadir. Then they will cycle out my own blood, clear out the leukemic cells and return healthy blood back to my body. This will then have my body ideally produce cancer-free blood going forward.

The other type of transplant is called an allogeneic transplant. With this we have to find a healthy person whose human leukocyte antigen (HLA) matches mine. Then their bone marrow will be taken from them and donated to me. That sounds simple right?

For me since my bone marrow is producing leukemic cancer cells, it is necessary for me to have the allogeneic cell transplant. Are you still with me? This means that first thing we will need to do is find someone who matches with me. This is so overwhelming, and I have a lot to learn. This is all information I have found out by asking the nurses and getting answers to questions that I ask good old GOOGLE. Remember how helpful Google has been.

To be a donor they must be an HLA match. HLAs are proteins that are in most cells in the human body. To be a donor they are looking for the donor to match 10 out of 10. The most likely matches are siblings and other family members. I only have 1 full brother, and I hope he is a match. If he doesn't match, or isn't able to donate, then my medical team will reach out to Be The Match (BTM), which is made up of millions of people from the world who have chosen to be registered to be a potential donor. Hopefully it doesn't come to that, so let's take this one step at a time.

Fortunately for me, my brother, Ben, just arrived back from 2 weeks in Europe. He has been following my journey over the past month and said he was 100% here for me if I needed anything. Now with that being said I'm not sure that he realized that being 100% there for me meant that I would be asking him to be tested to donate his stem cells to save my life. As soon as he arrived home, I asked if he would be willing to be tested to see if he was a match to be my donor. He said he is all in. He is my brother; I am so lucky. There is apparently a 25% chance that he could be a match. It would be incredible if he matched.

To find out if Ben is a match he have to get his blood drawn to do HLA matching and to see if Ben and my blood cells match. They have told me this could take awhile. What does awhile mean? Do I have awhile to wait? I keep getting mixed messages, and as you already know I'm not very patient. While we wait, I have to stop these bad blood cell from growing.

The oncology team presented me with a few options to try to get me into remission allowing me to have a clean slate before my BMT. The options are to redo the exact same chemo regimen that we just completed, 3 days of Idarubicin, and 7 days at 24 hours a day of Cytarabine. The second chemo option is a chemo called Fludarabine, and a very high dose of Cytarabine along with Neupogen shots to boost my white blood cells. All of the above options require that I remain in the hospital for a month again. To determine which of the above options I/we go with, they will need to have the bone marrow results back, so this puts me in another waiting period. Neither one of the chemo regimens sounds like fun but I guess I have to do one of them. The doctor said it was up to me which one I do. Seriously, up to me? How can I know which is better? I mean, the first one that I already did worked a bit but not all the way. Also, the reason I'm okay doing it again is it worked a lot. Not all of the way but it helped a lot. Also, I really didn't get a lot of side effects. I hear horrible things about what happens to people and really, I was lucky. The second chemo treatment is a good idea. Something new and maybe it will completely get rid of the cancer. That could really prepare my body for the BMT/SCT if I'm able to have it. What about the side effects from that one? Something new scares me. Putting all of these toxins in my body is awful, but then again cancer is awful for my body. So, shoot, what is best? I don't really have a lot of time to think about this. What is best to get me into remission?

Since I don't have a fever and my main ailment is my swollen achilles tendon and my sore mouth, my doctor told me that I might be able to go home for a few days during this waiting game. I would love that, even if all I do is sleep in my own bed and lay on my own couch; I want to go home.

As always, the highlight of my day was seeing my crazy kiddos and my husband. Alyssa made me a sun catcher for my window that is shaped like a butterfly so I can suction cup it to my window and think of her every time I look out my window. Eli pulled all of the snacks out of the snack cabinet and danced to the monkey on the iPad. It's always nice to be able to forget about what is going on for 30 minutes or an hour and enjoy the energy and sunshine that Eli and Alyssa bring. My family is why I am fighting this fight. They are what is keeping me going.

I guess this is the marathon that we talked about in the beginning. I'm continuing to run this and appreciate everyone's support as I keep fighting this fight. Obviously, I'm not happy about this latest update, but I also am a bit numb right now. I'm just focusing on whatever I need to do to move forward. We are looking at a possible second opinion with a leukemia specialist at Stanford. We obviously can't do anything until we have all of the necessary information, but once we get more detailed information by the end of this week, early next week we will be able to get that second opinion.

August 1, 2013
A LITTLE SOMETHING TO LOOK FORWARD TO...

FINALLY! Yesterday's news was certainly not what any of us were looking forward to. After having some time to think it through, and really realize what lies ahead, I am ready for the next challenge, and look forward to kicking leukemia to the curb with this next treatment.

I'm trying to not get too excited, but the doctor said that as long as nothing crazy happened today (meaning no fever etc.) and tonight, then I can go home tomorrow for a few days. I am super excited and look forward to getting off the third floor of the hospital. I have been detached from my IV pole, and things are looking promising.

Alyssa and Eli spent the night at Grandma and Papa's for the second time last night. Uncle Ben and his fiancée Cody helped take care of them, and they did great (both the kids, and all of the adults). The kids had so much fun, and Alyssa told me all about her awesome slumber party with them when she came to visit today.

The nurse came to weigh me today, which turned into everyone in the family including Ben and Cody getting weighed. We are all doing well on our weight. I've not gained any more weight but not lost any, so I'll take that as a good thing. Dave and I had some time today to play cards, however we were disappointed to realize that we don't remember how to play many games. We tried to play Speed, however I'm not sure what version we ended up playing, because it was not right. We will have to brush up on our card playing before my next hospital stay.

Everyone's responses to yesterday's bad news was so appreciated. Many people mentioned interest in donating bone marrow and how we could find out if any of you were a match. The easiest way to get on the registry is to go to the link below.

http://bethematch.org/Join/Join_the_Registry.aspx

They are accepting potential donors ages 18-40. It is really easy to log in online and answer some questions. When you are approved to be a donor, they will mail you a kit to swab the inside of your mouth. It is simple. There are two long Q-Tips, and you swab the inside of each of your cheeks. Then you send it back and they put your name on an international registry. If you know anyone who would be interested in being registered, please spread the word.

There are also bone marrow drives that are done often so you can see if there is a bone marrow drive in your area coming up that you can get swabbed to get on the registry.

You know how I said it was ironic that I used to donate blood and now I need blood? Well, you aren't going to believe this. Immediately after college I had moved back home and was asked by a doctor at UCSF to help him with his research. He needed people to donate bone marrow to better understand how healthy marrow could help with blood disorders. I thought sure, I'm all about research. I'd be happy to donate. After that I became so interested in how bone marrow could help people, so a group of friends and I worked with the Red Cross and ran a bone marrow drive at UC Berkeley. During that we registered a bunch of potential donors. I even got myself on the bone marrow registry. Now here I am 20 years later, and I am benefiting from all of that research. Now if that isn't ironic, I don't know what is.

I'm excited to offer updates from my home for the next couple days. Wishing everyone a wonderful Friday, as always, I'm excited to hear what everyone is up to this weekend.

AUGUST 2, 2013

I was so excited that I might be able to go home today. I packed up my room, and when Dave came in at 9:30 a.m. he started loading up the car. Apparently, all of the excitement definitely wore me out, because I was ready for a nap by 11 a.m. When my doctor came in to let me know my next steps, the doctor told me that even if Ben is a match, it will take 10+ days to determine that. They keep changing the time frame, but I am just excited things are in process. Since it will take so long for the potential transplant to start even if Ben is a match, Dr. S is not comfortable holding off any chemo treatment any later than Friday, August 9.

Meanwhile, in the last few days, I have been able to get an appointment for a second opinion with the AML specialist at Stanford. I will see him next Wednesday when I am home and get some ideas of what a good treatment for me would be.

While we wait for the Stanford doctor to share their thoughts of what to do, and or for August 9 to come around. Dr. S finally told me exactly what I've wanted to hear for ages. He discharged me and told me to go home for some much-earned R&R. Even better, I don't have to return until Friday the 9th. Obviously, I am ecstatic. It felt like an eternity waiting for the paperwork to be done and for the pharmacy to get my meds ready. Oh, the pharmacy, it is unbelievable how many medications I came home with. Fortunately, the pharmacist went over each one with me, and many of the meds are ones that I've been taking every day since I've been in the hospital, which was 34 days by the way (but who's counting).

It's difficult because part of me always imagined that when I came home, I would be in remission, so I don't like the idea that I'm not in remission or done with chemo. Overall, I don't care, it is so wonderful to be out of the hospital. I felt like I was breaking the rules as I got on the elevator and walked out of the hospital. I have not been out of the third floor for over a month. Isn't that crazy? I don't think I've ever been in a place for that long before. The exit that I left through is one that I had never been through before (I had only come through the ER in the past).

Every day from my room I was able to watch Dave and the kids enter and exit the hospital for their visits. Today I was actually able to see where they walked every day, and what they were able to see up in my room when I waved at them. It was so bizarre, I hadn't been in an elevator, in a car, etc. for 34 days. When we pulled in the driveway of our house, Alyssa came running out and was so excited to see me. She didn't even want to be separated from me for a second. She wanted to show me everything. While I was gone Alyssa learned how to pump on the swings. Up until now we've had to push her when she wants to play on the swings, but we won't have to do that anymore. She was so proud of herself, and I was so proud of her. Eli seemed to be excited that I was home and was excited to sit in the wagon so I could pull her around the patio. She also showed me her new skill of toilet diving. She looks into the toilet and tries to put her hand in it. Gross. Now I understand why there is a baby lock on our toilets. Brady (our fur baby), on the other hand, showed little interest in me, probably because he knows I didn't come home to take him for a walk.

Even though I didn't get home until 2:15 p.m. today, those 5 hours while the kids were awake were wonderful and absolutely exhausting. Alyssa didn't want to leave my side, and we read books, played outside, had snacks, ate dinner together, and did art projects. In some ways it felt like we were cramming in as much as we could while we could. I look forward to hanging out for the next couple days, enjoying being at home with the family before my next month in the hospital. I know I'm not supposed to think ahead, but I am thinking about it, and I am scared of what is to come next. I wish everyone a wonderful weekend full of fun.

AUGUST 3, 2013
HOME FOR A WHOLE DAY!

It was so wonderful to sleep in my own bed last night. I slept pretty well and really did enjoy being home. There were no nurses coming in to wake me up in the middle of the night for my vitals etc. The kids both slept great, and I was able to sleep in until 6:30 a.m. We enjoyed a fun/chaotic breakfast together in person. No worrying about the internet going out, or the computer being dropped. I got to eat whatever I wanted, whenever I wanted meaning, I wasn't on the hospital's meal delivery schedule. It is the little things that I'm learning to appreciate. The bummer is that all of these things totally wore me out, so I had to take a nap at 8 a.m.

One of the awesome things that happened while I was in the hospital is that my family redid the shed in our backyard. We have a 13' by 18' shed in the backyard that previously was the man lair. It was unfinished on the sides and had a roll up garage door on the front facing the yard. I never knew why it was built that way, but it must have made sense to the previous owner. It had housed a Ping-Pong table, a dart board, our earthquake supplies, along with a handful of black widows. We always joked that if there was an earthquake we would go to the shed to get our earthquake supplies and get bit by a black widow. I'm not sure if that made sense.

That is no longer a worry, now the shed has been transformed into the "cottage." It is almost done and is beautiful. The roll-up garage door has been replaced by beautiful French doors. There is a desk, 2 bookshelves and an electric fireplace. It also has a great futon. This is bigger and so much more beautiful than that first hospital room I was in. This will be my office when I go back to work and will also be a great place where I can relax when I am home between chemo treatments. It still needs some finishing touches but is a fantastic addition to our house. Now I just have to be home more to enjoy it!

I stayed home all day; I got to go outside and enjoy the sun while watching the kids play. Without overdoing it I plan to go walk to the park just down the street tomorrow. Overall, I have been feeling really good; the only pain I have is a little bit in my mouth, and then the area where they did the biopsy on the back of my pelvic bone is very tender and swollen. That is to be expected, the best way I can explain it is a bad bruise. Overall though I feel great; I'm definitely enjoying my time here. It was funny at lunch time today I was eating my soup, and Alyssa said, "Mommy, aren't you supposed to take medicine with your lunch?" Um, yep, she was right, I was forgetting my medicine. Thank goodness I have her to keep me in line and on top of my meds.

Today was the day we had booked our family trip to Maine. Since we couldn't be there, we brought the Maine experience to my parents' house for dinner. Lobster, corn, popovers, and family time. It's not exactly the same as being in Maine, but it certainly was an awesome substitute considering the circumstances. As much as I try to forget all that is going on with my health, it is still present. The way it sunk into me the most was at dinner. I'm not a huge fan of lobster. I know I sound very snotty. The thing is, I don't like getting the meat out of the shell; it is too messy. As we were sitting down at the dinner table, my dad kindly took my lobster, cracked it in half. Took the lobster cracking tools and carefully used the forks to take all of the meat out of its shell. I sat there at my seat with my lobster bib on and tried my best to hold back the tears as they welled up in my eyes. It triggered something in me. I have always been a strong independent woman. My family always knew this about me, and people rarely did things for me. Here my dad was preparing my dinner for me: shelling my lobster... prepping the plate. Whether it was intentional or not, it looked to me like I needed help. He was feeding me like a baby (a baby who eats lobster). I'm his daughter and he needs to take care of me. I was no longer the independent woman I had always been. I think I held it together but inside I was falling apart. We had such a fun day, but I have to admit hanging out at home even though I'm laying low is exhausting. Looking forward to more wonderful exhausting days ahead before I move back into Kaiser.

AUGUST 4, 2013
LET THE GOOD TIMES ROLL

I had another great night at home. I still woke up once or twice during the night, probably because that is what I've been trained to do, but I still slept well. I actually think I fell asleep on the couch last night before 9 p.m. Things seemed a lot less chaotic this morning, it is as if I'm getting back into the routine. Don't get me wrong, Dave still does the bulk of the work in the mornings. He gets up with the kids, takes the dog out, gets breakfast done; he really has things down (isn't he incredible?). I love that I get to eat real food when I want it and I don't have to wait for it to be brought to my room or served to me.

I was so excited to take my first shower at home, since I have this central line in my chest, I have to be super careful that I don't get the line wet. At the hospital they taught me how to tape everything up before I take a shower. Well apparently, I wasn't as good of a student as I had thought, because somehow the taping job I did was completely ineffective, and I ended up getting the dressing and the lines completely soaking wet. If this line didn't go straight into my heart, I might not have been as worried, but since it does, I had to call the advice line and they told me to go to the ER to get the dressing changed. Here I was, after only 1 full day out of the hospital, I had to go visit again. Fortunately, it was just for a quick 1-hour trip to the ER to get my dressing changed. In the future, I guess I will leave the taping to the professionals until I get a better handle on it.

After we returned home from the ER, I enjoyed and afternoon of fun with the kiddos and was able to even take advantage of quiet time. It is amazing what a difference it is to be home. Even if all I was doing was taking it easy. I was sitting on my couch, walking outside, breathing the fresh air when I wanted to. I know this sounds so simple, but I hadn't done this for over a month. Playing with my kids when I wanted to. Sitting on the floor having all of their toys. Going to the refrigerators and getting food when I wanted to. Getting water in my cup. Heating up food in the microwave whenever I wanted to. Shoot even doing dishes at my sink. This all sounds so trivial but it isn't. These are simple things that I wasn't able to do for so long. There really is so much to appreciate about the comforts of your own home. We had a delicious dinner of steak, veggies and farro; even Alyssa ate the farro. I've decided my goal is to pack on the pounds while I'm home. It won't be hard; the food is so good. It is also healthy and not processed. I continue to be perplexed that the food in the hospital seems to be so bad for you. It is all processed and canned or overall not good for you. I love that while at home I can really eat whatever I want whenever I want. I don't have to wait for specific times for it to be delivered and to have to choose from crappy food.

Our family has always talked about our highs and lows at dinner time. You know mentioning the best and worst things that happened during your day? Well, tonight we all agreed that the highlight of the day was having me home. It makes it that much harder to know that I have to go back to the hospital soon, but it will be okay. We got the kiddos off to bed, and Dave and I just enjoyed being together.

AUGUST 5, 2013
ANOTHER UNPLANNED TWIST

I enjoyed another great night at home in my own bed. Have I mentioned this enough? I woke up in the middle of the night and noticed pain and swelling in my left foot. To help it I slept with my foot up on pillows to reduce the swelling. I think this is similar to my swollen Achilles tendon the other day, so I just continue to ice it and keep it raised when I can. I'm not sure if this is something random that is just my body's way of acting or is it something I need to worry about more?

I had my first outpatient appointment today to get my blood drawn. The appointment was at 7:30 a.m., and it was a bit tough to get both kids, Dave, and I out the door on time. It was rough going in to get my blood drawn. I need to realize that this is my new life, this is going to be part of my outpatient life. My foot was still swollen (much less than it was last night) but still swollen so I brought it up to the nurse. She drew my blood and called the doctor, since she was a bit concerned. She thought that the swollen foot could be a blood clot. That meant a 5-minute appointment for just the blood draw turned out to be a lot longer. In hindsight I'm wondering if I should have played down the swelling since it had reduced from last night and it could be nothing. At the same time, every little thing makes me nervous. It is a catch. I don't want to make a big deal about things because I want to be at home as long as I can. Then at the same time, what if I ignore it and it is really a big deal? Really what is the best thing to do? Well, it is too late, I already told the nurse, and I'm sure they are doing the best thing for me health wise.

After Dr. S looked at my foot, he was concerned about an infection and felt that it was in my best interest to get admitted to the hospital. This was very upsetting. Here we had rushed the whole family together with planned plans for a quick trip to the ER, and hopefully a day together, and now it was no longer a fun family day but a scary complete change of plans. I really wanted the kids to keep thinking the hospital was a fun place. I had said I would be home for a few days. This meant that my 2.5 days of home time bliss was now over, and I was going to be in the hospital for a month again.

Not only was I not prepared with all of the packing I had to do, mentally I was not here at all. I was and still am devastated by this. Here I had planned on a few days with the family, I was in control of what I could eat, who I could see, where I could sleep and now it was all out of my control again. Although I went with it, and I am learning this is what I need to do. Just go with what happens, live in the moment. This was very difficult for me. It really took everything in me not to throw a huge tantrum to show how mad, sad, and frustrated I was with this. This cancer has created this new life that me and my family now had to live with. This isn't fair. Oh, such an easy thing to say and yet, it isn't fair. No one should have to live this way, but here we are, trying to figure it out.

Since we had planned on this being a quick appointment, we had the whole family with us. This meant that the whole family had to go to the ER, to get me through triage, and into an ER bed while we waited for a room on the third floor. Alyssa was a trooper while we waited, it helped that there was a TV in the ER room, and they had plenty of snacks for the kids. It took a few hours before they were able to get me out of the ER, and fortunately in that time my mom was able to come get the kids, so it was just Dave and me in the little ER room. They started me on IV antibiotics to combat any infection that may be causing the swelling. I have learned that IV antibiotics is the quick response to anything when they don't know what is causing my pain or swelling. Normally I would push back, as I'm not a fan of antibiotics and I like to be educated about what medications are being put in my body, but since I am so immuno-compromised and my body is so fragile, I will accept anything they are giving me. Shoot, I've had a month with chemo killing my body, and I'm about to do it again. I guess I will let them do anything to keep me going. As the antibiotics were being administered and slowly dripped through the IV. A room became available, and I was moved upstairs around noon.

I was bummed to learn that my penthouse suite was occupied by another patient, but I was moved into a double room with a great big window and a good view. This room has 2 beds, and since I'm neutropenic I don't have a roommate. This worked out well for Dave; he made himself at home in the other bed. As I type this, he is actually sleeping in his own hospital bed. I better be careful; the nurses may start thinking he is the patient and give him the medications.

I'm coming to terms with the fact that I'm back in the hospital for 4 more weeks. I really had a great time being at home, and I loved that I got to spend the time that I did with Dave, the kids, and the rest of the family at our house. I also had some fantastic food which was great. I really feel that I took advantage of my time at home, so although I wish I could have had more time, I know I made the most of it. I find these unplanned changes in schedule are very diffi-cult for me, but once I have time for it to soak in, I am better able to accept that this is what is happening, and that it really is best for me in the long run even though it is tough to have changes that are not what I want. I find that it is most important for me to find the posi-tives in all of these moments or else I would be drowning in the challenges that I am immersed in. The more I find the positives the easier it is for me to keep moving forward. As I continue to think about how difficult this is for me, I can't even begin to imagine how hard this is for the rest of my family. All of the plans and logistics that are constantly in flux. As hard as I feel all of this is for me, they really have it hard.

One positive thing about being here now is that I can start my next round of chemo earlier then I had planned. I have a second opinion scheduled at Stanford on Wednesday, but now that I can't go physically, they want to cancel the appointment. I will need to speak with them to understand if I can still have the appointment or how that would work. Ideally my parents could go, and I could be there over FaceTime. I will know more tomorrow after I speak with their office.

It's only 7 p.m., but I'm exhausted. My life has become an emotional rollercoaster and today went from high to low. The kids have been awesome and are spending the night at my parents' house, which gives Dave some much needed downtime and also allows the kids some fun time away. The kids do well with my parents when they are there for the night which has been a savior these last couple weeks. Now that I'm back in the hospital I have more time to respond to emails again, so keep them coming, keep the fun weekend stories coming. I really thrive being able to live vicariously through you.

It is great to hear what everyone is up to and how everyone is doing. Living vicariously through you all is fantastic and keeps me going.

AUGUST 6, 2013
ONWARD AND UPWARD

I miss my great nights of sleep from my time at home. It is far from smooth here. It didn't help that they were changing out my IV antibiotics at midnight and 1 a.m. Luckily, I can sleep through it all pretty well. They also wake me up at 6 for more IV antibiotics and to do the daily blood draw. Even though I know this was my routine for over a month, I seemed to have trouble adjusting to it today. My left foot is still swollen but less red. We haven't received any update on the cultures, so we do not know if it is an actual infection or not.

The kids came by this morning and were here briefly; they found great joy in playing hide and seek with the little built-in closet in my room. They are such goof balls! Alyssa and Dave went to the movies together. They have found a theater that is geared towards kids in the summer and plays movies on Tuesday and Wednesday mornings. This has become their weekly father-daughter activity over the last few weeks.

I called Stanford today about my appointment tomorrow to see if I could get a second opinion even if I wasn't physically there. My parents were going to go and then I planned on being available over face time or another HIPAA compliant solution so they could see that I'm not wasting away but am still a vibrant young woman just trying to kick this AML to the curb. Unfortunately, they will not do a second opinion without having me be physically there. It boggles my mind that with a diagnosis such as AML where time is not on my side, that they are not open to alternative ways of handling second opinions. It seems to me that since 95% of the second opinion is dependent on numbers and paperwork and really only 5% requires actually seeing me, it is ridiculous to me that they wouldn't make this accommodation. I realize I'm a bit biased because I have worked in telemedicine for the last 3 years before I was diagnosis with leukemia. I know it is available in a HIPPAA compliant manner. This is a perfect example of where it could be put to use. I'm sure I could argue it more, but I'm not sure it is worth it since I am trying to be on their good side.

Anyway, that saves my parents a trip to Stanford which is about 60 miles away which can take anywhere from 60 minutes to 3 hours just to drive there one way. In addition, Dr. M, the AML Stanford oncologist, and my Kaiser oncology team had recommended a treatment called GCLAC for this round of chemo. This is a sister treatment to the more common FLAG treatment that my oncologist uses more often. Knowing they had talked took the pressure off of me having to determine what path I would take.

With that, we decided that we would move forward as soon as possibly with the GCLAC treatment that they agreed on. They ordered the chemo, and it won't be available until Wednesday night, so instead of getting me prepped to start chemo today we will begin the prep tomorrow. The way this round will work is, I will begin getting Neupogen tomorrow. This will help build my white blood cell count. Then approximately 24 hours after the Neupogen has begun they will start the chemo. This treatment will be 5 days long receiving the chemo a few hours each day in a highly concentrated dose. I will know much more about this once it starts, so I will bore you with more details later. The Neupogen has been known to cause pain in the bones and joints, so it is helpful to know what to expect and be ready for what may come. Otherwise, the chemo treatment should have similar side effects to the previous chemo.

My biggest concern last time was losing my hair, now I actually welcome losing the rest of my hair since I have an odd group of stragglers that I'd be happy to bid farewell to. I'd look like Gollum in *Lord of the Rings* if I hadn't shaved my hair. I spent the rest of the day walking around the hospital floor, trying to eat as much as possible, and my biggest accomplishment of the day was a call with the DMV (how often can you say that?). Yes, that a positive experience was a call with the DMV. My license expired last month, and I had renewed it, however, when I was admitted last time, in all the confusion of moving in, somehow Dave and I misplaced my brand-new license. The DMV has a wonderful policy that if you need a new license not only do you have to make an appointment, go to the DMV, and pay the additional fee, but you also have to take a new photo without a hat, and that will be your photo for the next 5 years. Although I have had many unflattering ID photos, and I am very accepting of my balding head, I am not ready to have my license picture be one of me in the middle of chemo. Fortunately, after waiting for the DMV to call me back 2 hours after I called them (thank goodness for the call back feature), I was connected with someone who said he would issue me a new license and send it in the mail. This means I don't have to go there in person, and I don't have to get a new photo taken for another 5 or more years. Phew! I love that things are going much easier than I anticipated today. I hope that is an omen for how things will keep going throughout this treatment.

We have been so overwhelmed with everyone's support. I have accepted that I'm back in the hospital earlier than planned, yet I've spent the day in and out of tears so overwhelmed with everyone's generosity with their time, love, prayers, thoughts, meals, dog walks, etc. I always knew we had amazing people in our life, but everyone has just astonished me with how they have involved themselves in our life to help us get through this together. I can never thank everyone enough but want to let you know your love and support is truly felt by our whole family.

AUGUST 8, 2013
WEDNESDAY'S UPDATE LAST NIGHT

Last night I had the LVN who likes to come in and have a conversation at 12:30 a.m. or 1 a.m. when he takes my vitals. You have got to be kidding me. Do I look like I want to be woken up to have a conversation in the middle of the night? Well, I don't. Fortunately, he got the hint when I closed my eyes and rolled over away from him.

Overall, I had a nice day, nothing disastrous happened, which in my opinion, makes it a pretty fantastic day. You are probably wondering how my foot is doing, well, it's still swollen, but doesn't really hurt and doesn't seem red. All of the cultures have come back negative so they are thinking this may just be swelling related to the chemo.

The kiddos did their usual visit. We walked around the third floor and gave Eli a chance to stretch her legs and continue to take a few steps. It is so funny, I don't remember Alyssa taking so long from when she did her first steps to when she was really off and walking, but maybe my memory is playing tricks on me (now I know why people keep baby books). Alyssa hung out with me for a few hours on her own. She was loving sitting in Dave's bed, yes now everyone has their own bed in the room in the hospital. She loved watching tv and ordering snacks from the nurse. Today cherry Jell-O was her snack of choice. It was fun to cuddle and watch kids shows with her.

I received some good news today. The preliminary results have come back from the bone marrow matching, and it looks like Ben and I are a match. WAHOO! This is the best news ever. They are doing further testing, but this is looking great so far. I started Neupogen today, the new chemo hasn't arrived at the hospital yet so I'm hoping to start it tomorrow, but we are not sure if that would be possible. As the day went on about 8 hours after receiving the Neupogen, I started to feel the discomfort that they warned me about. It feels like growing pains in my hips and knees, so they gave me Claritin to reduce the discomfort. Hoping the Claritin will help relieve the discomfort. That seems so odd to me that an allergy medicine can help relieve bone pain. I don't know how they figured that out, but I'm glad they did. I didn't get started on writing this until later than usual, so I will keep it short. Have a wonderful evening!

AUGUST 8, 2013
CHEMO DAY 1 OF 5 BEGINS!

I'm getting used to being woken up many, many times at night; it is just how things are here, and it looks like they will be keeping me on antibiotics for 7-14 days even if there is no infection.

The chemo finally arrived, and I started it this afternoon, which was somewhat anticlimactic. I'm excited to have started it though so I can get these 5 days going. They gave me the Neupogen again this morning. Although I need it to help build my white blood cells. The pain it caused in my bones throughout my body is awful. This time even the Claritin didn't help reduce the pain. I'm trying to massage my legs and do some other things to try to reduce the discomfort.

I had the usual fun visit with the kids, Alyssa wanted to cuddle in bed and color. Oh, how I love this. She drew her first picture for me for my new room. Eli as usual kind of finds her way around the room and is mostly interested in me when there is food involved. Both kids have learned to request food from the nurses here, so they are well fed after their visits.

I meant to mention yesterday how proud I was about all the food I consumed. I have an appetite and am able to eat pretty well right now, so I've been taking advantage of it. Yesterday I ate a whole small/medium pizza, chicken soup, half a cheeseburger, and pasta. I was so impressed with myself. This is a huge improvement in my food consumption, going from eating a little soup here and there to eating this enormous smorgasbord of food. I'm hoping to be able to keep it up so I don't stop being able to eat and lose so much weight if the chemo makes it hard for me to eat or keep food down. We had a fun full-on family picnic dinner tonight. We all enjoyed different foods with plenty for everyone to enjoy. We had so much fun.

I was also able to take a nap today which doesn't happen often because people are constantly coming in and out of my room. I may be getting a Do Not Disturb sign for the door like in hotels. They do not offer that, but it sure would be nice. I'm hoping the internet lets me post this in a more timely manner tonight. Hope everyone's week is going well and that you have a great weekend ahead of you.

AUGUST 9, 2013
CHEMO DAY 2 OF 5. BRING IT ON!

My leg cramps/restless leg syndrome didn't bother me while I was sleeping last night which was great. I think I fell asleep right around 9 p.m. I did experience some nausea around 11 p.m. I learned that if I ask for nausea medication along with a bucket, they bring the medication really quickly! Isn't that funny?

Today was the day that I was supposed to be readmitted to start chemo; I guess I wanted to get a jump on it and come in early, right? My foot, which I blame for my early admission to the hospital on Monday, is no longer swollen, so I was relieved to learn that I can be off IV antibiotics. This means they won't be bugging me at midnight and 1 a.m. to change my IVs. It also means I can sleep without being connected to the IV pump. Unfortunately, as things seem to go here, moments later I was informed that as part of the treatment I need to be on 24/7 saline drip. NOOOOOOO! For some reason it drives me nuts to be attached to the darn IV pole, I know you heard enough of it with the last chemo treatments but come on!! I just love freedom. Okay… vent over, I'll accept it, and deal with it for the next 3 days.

Dave and Eli came to visit me nice and early this morning, and we were joined by Alyssa a bit later. Eli had fun playing with some finger puppets with different jungle animals. That kept her occupied for a while. In a proud parenting moment, Eli wanted a sharpened pencil to play with, and I chose to give her a pen instead thinking it was the safer option. However, she managed to take it apart and tear it into at least 6 pieces in a matter of seconds. I guess I should be thankful that she didn't break into the ink, and when Alyssa came later, she was able to put it back together. I guess I will be recalling my application for mother of the year.

We also realized today that possibly the reason that Eli was a bit cranky last week was because she got a new tooth that I noticed today; it's pretty much halfway in. Alyssa got to stay with me for a while so we could enjoy some time together, just her and me, after Eli and Dave left. I'm so glad we can make the most of the little time we have together.

The only real side effects I am feeling today are the restless legs from the Neupogen, and then I find myself more tired than usual and have a bit of nausea. One of the medications that I'm on was the same one I was on before but instead of having it delivered over 24 hours I am receiving the same dose over 2 hours which I think increases the side effects of exhaustion. With that being said I wouldn't be surprised if I go to bed by 9 most nights. I also started a new medication to try to relieve the restless legs so hopefully that does the trick.

Hope everyone has had a great Friday and is looking forward to a fun weekend. As always, I look forward to hearing your plans for this fun filled weekend.

AUGUST 10, 2013
CHEMO DAY 3 OF 5. LOOPY DEE DOO!

Today has been my toughest day pain wise so far. I woke up at 2 a.m. with what I thought was indigestion; I was able to have some hot water and go back to sleep. I woke up again at 5 a.m. in excruciating pain that I again thought was indigestion. When I would try to take deep breaths to relax, it actually was worse because it increased the pain. We spent much of the day trying to understand what was going on. In the early afternoon my mom brought up the idea that this could actually be bone pain. I have been icing it, and also taking pain medications that should help. Once we figured out that it could be sternum pain caused by the Neupogen, the nurse mentioned using an injectable morphine medication called Dilaudid. The nurse got it approved and they injected it into my line. I don't know how to explain it, but the feeling was incredible. All of a sudden, I felt a rush come through my body and within 30 seconds the pain was gone, and I felt incredible. Now other than the drugs that I've been taking at the hospital I've not taken drugs recreationally, but I completely understand it now. It felt great and the pain was completely gone. They can only give that to me every couple hours as needed. Fortunately, that one time was enough to get me through the day.

Fortunately, the kids came for their daily visit after the pain was gone. Alyssa is very interested in having more mommy and me time, I'm hoping once we get into more of a schedule with Dave going back to work, we can find some time to do that. I'm pretty tired today so I am going to keep today's update short. I'm looking forward to learning more about ways to help relieve the pain in the easiest way possible. The pain meds make me loopy and unable to concentrate, so I'm going to call it a night, before this gets really interesting.

AUGUST 11, 2013
CHEMO DAY 4 OF 5 AND DOING GREAT

Yesterday was definitely rough, but today was miles better. I still have the bone pain in my sternum, but knowing that it is bone pain and not indigestion has really helped me focus on what the issue is and medicate appropriately. I continued to take the Dilaudid at night but was able to switch to Norco during the day, which is much better since it doesn't make me so loopy. It made it hard to read my updates as I was typing them, so it is nice today to actually be able to read what I'm typing and feel like I'm slightly more coherent than I was yesterday. I actually was up at 4:30 a.m. for the day, which meant I took my first nap at 8 a.m.

Dave brought the kids by, and Eli continued to show off her walking. It has been so funny how hesitant she has been wanting to walk. She keeps seeming like she's ready to walk more on her own and gets more confident, and then she realizes how much more quickly she can crawl and goes back to just crawling. Both kids showed up today in Adidas sweat suits. It was so cute; they looked ready to work out.

I completed the 4th of 5 chemo treatments today, one more day of chemo before the waiting game begins. I'm hoping to keep some of these updates short (That means less drama which is a very good thing). Oh, I also got word that my old hospital penthouse room may be available tomorrow. Although I really like my current room, I prefer to have the double doors like I did before. It gives me a little privacy with the decontamination room for people to wash their hands and everything before they come in. It also decreases the number of people that just walk into the room from all of the cleaning people and the multiple trash pick ups. Fingers crossed I get to go back to my old room. This round of chemo knocks me out, so I am going to bed much earlier than I was before (Probably also explains why I'm up at 4 a.m.). Have a great week!

AUGUST 12, 2013
CHEMO DAY 5 COMPLETE!

I had another good day; I hope these keep going in the right direction. I went to bed really early last night and was up from 2 a.m.-3:15 a.m. just hanging out. I had asked my nurse to wake me up with pain pills every 4 hours to keep me ahead of the pain curve. However when they came in at 2:15 a.m. I didn't have any pain; it was awesome.

I also apparently decided that I had a major craving for a chocolate peanut butter shake from Jamba Juice. Since I knew that Dave wouldn't be woken up by a text, I felt just fine sending my request at this ungodly hour and that he would see it in the morning. I was able to go back to sleep and then dream of it for the rest of the night.

Today was day 5 of 5 for my latest round of chemo. This is very exciting. To celebrate, I wore my Super Man shirt (much to Alyssa's delight). This also meant that by the end of the day I could be detached from the IV pole and walk around free again. This time I've been attached to a very high-tech pole (just because it came with the room), so it has an oxygen tank, and is twice as wide to walk with. It basically means that I walk into a lot of walls when I'm out and about, and I often run into the doors around the room. The hospital will be a much safer place once I get separated from this pole. I'm looking forward to my big walk around the hospital tomorrow without my buddy.

I got to FaceTime with the kids at breakfast this morning before they had their first day with their new babysitter. They both seem excited and ready to have a great day. We will be switching up our routine, so instead of the kids visiting in the morning, they will have to start visiting in the afternoon/evening, since Dave will be back at work. It will be a change, but part of the new deal allows Alyssa to visit the hospital in her jammies, and Eli seemed to be quite content hanging out after dinner. Dave brought the delicious Jamba Juice milkshake I was craving. Yeah, for 2 a.m. cravings that are still delicious hours later.

Other than finishing my 5th day of treatment (which is pretty monumental) my day was pretty chill. Now the waiting game begins again. The goal is to keep me in the hospital until 28 days post chemo treatment. I'm optimistic that if I can stay healthy again this time, I can make it home before the 28-day biopsy.

I am still hoping to switch rooms but found out that I missed my chance to go to the penthouse suite yesterday. Doh, I'm super bummed, but I will stick with my current double room. They also are hot to have me switch rooms because right now my room has me taking up 2 beds when they would much prefer I be in a room with a single bed. As I mentioned yesterday, things may be a bit boring as we go through the next 23 days. Remember, boring is good regarding any additional health issues, but I know some of the side effects will start coming on soon. Wishing everyone a great evening and a fantastic week ahead.

AUGUST 13, 2013
WAITING WITH PLENTY OF ENERGY

I had a new nurse for the night shift, and she had asked if I was ambulatory and needed any help with getting to the bathroom at night. I let her know I was fine and could hold my own. Fast forward to 4 a.m. I woke up and called my nurse to see if she could get me a pain med, and a Boost (the supplement that I enjoy drinking in the middle of the night). Sure enough, she walks in the room with a second nurse, I thought, wow I certainly asked for 2 things, but didn't think it required a second nurse. Turns out she had thought that when I asked for a Boost, I was asking to be lifted up in the bed instead of just wanting a drink. It was pretty funny, and I'm sure it was all the talk of the night staff! At least I hope that was the only drama they had that night.

My days continue to go well, I actually just realized that I have been on a steroid meds for the last couple days so now that I'm not attached to the pole anymore, I feel like Magda from *There's Something About Mary* (though with a bit less vigor, and much less of a tan) where I just want to run around, and tackle any and all projects. If you don't know what I'm talking about, you have to watch the movie and you will totally get it.

I was offered a room with double doors today right next to my old penthouse suite. I got quite excited and went to check it out. Thank goodness they let me approve it before moving me. The room had a bed, 3 chairs, an IV pole, and a closet, and I don't know if I would have been able to even walk around the bed if I was in there. It was so small. I think it is smaller than my very first room was. I like that there was a great view of the trees, but it was really dark, and all I could think of was that if I had to be in that room for 22 more days, I would go insane. Let's keep me to one wild diagnosis at a time. They are thinking that I may be able to move into the penthouse suite over the weekend. Isn't it funny that I'm calling a room in the hospital a penthouse? I felt bad not accepting it, and really the room I have now is HUGE, but apparently my sanity is more important than being in double door isolation.

The kids came this evening, and I have to say I like this new evening routine. Not only do I get to see the kids in the evening, but they bring delicious dinner with them, so I don't have to rely on my horrible hospital meals. All of you amazing people in our village are bringing us meal after meal, which is not only feeding Dave and the kids, but he is generously bringing it to me so we can enjoy it together. I have always enjoyed meals together, and it doesn't really matter where it is as long as it is together. I am stuffed to the gills and just hope I can sleep being so full.

We got to go play outside with the kids. I realize I hadn't really been outside in a week; it was fun to not only be out there, but also get to kick the ball around with Alyssa. Now outside is just a third floor cement area surrounded by the hospital walls, but hey, it is outside, somewhat clean air so I will take it. We played a little soccer, Eli walked from planter to planter, and Alyssa and I had a little sing off of the song, "Anything you can do I can do better." It is so fun. We compete, and she really is quite good at it. Shoot, she may be doing some things better than me.

I'm looking forward to a continued week of low numbers, and a wiped-out immune system. Hope everyone's weeks continue to go well.

AUGUST 14, 2013
FEELING GREAT WHILE I CONTINUE TO WAIT!

Last night was yet another night where my obsession with food has taken over. I had a great dinner last night with a delicious blueberry crumble dessert that I was too full to eat but was obsessed with. I decided that since I was so full I would plan on having it for breakfast at 6 a.m. It brought back memories of my favorite breakfast ever. Once we went on a trip to Oregon when I must have been less than 10 years old. We stayed with some people who didn't have children and they let me have blueberry pie with banana ice cream for breakfast. I remember thinking that was the best thing ever. Clearly my food obsession has not waned. I went to bed at 10 p.m. last night, and when I was woken up by the night nurse for my vitals, I was convinced it was 6 a.m. I couldn't believe they respected my wishes knowing how much I would appreciate a good night's sleep. Well turns out it wasn't 6 a.m., it was 12. They did my vitals, and I went back to bed. Finally, at 3 a.m., I couldn't help it anymore. I was wide awake and went straight to the fridge for the blueberry crumble. It was fantastic. I inhaled it and stayed up for an hour and a bit reading and enjoying some of the remaining part of the crumble, and the leftover steroid high. Even though I was up and hungry off and on all night, I was still able to be awake and enjoy my day.

The on-call oncologist still doesn't have any update on whether Ben continues to be a perfect match. I did learn that right now my white blood cell count is about as low as it can get. I may remain super low until it begins to pick up again in the coming days and once it hits a predetermined amount (2,000 Neutrophils) then I will be able to stop the Neupogen shots. Thank goodness, I have not been having any more side effects from the Neupogen. There has been no more restless legs, and the Claritin that I'm on seems to be keeping the pain in my sternum at bay. I did have a random situation this afternoon where I had a sudden sharp pain in my sternum that would not let go, the pain released quickly, but I still requested a pain med just to make sure I could stay ahead of the pain. It has not been an issue since.

The kids came after dinner tonight, and Alyssa and I partook in a fun art project. Of course it was great! It included sparkles which is always a win for all of us. I love sparkles, just not at home. She also made a great glitter glue drawing for me. The kids have been home with the new sitter during the day since Monday and things seem to be going great. Alyssa is definitely testing the babysitter, but she is being put in her place and boundaries are being established. It is tough for me to know that the kids can't be back in their preschool environment with their friends, but this is one of the many sacrifices that we need to take right now to make sure we keep the kids as healthy as possible and the germs out of our house. Eli attempted to couch dive and learned that that is not a good option for her. Luckily, she didn't get really hurt. I hope that she doesn't do that again. Eli has also proven to be a bit more curious than Alyssa was and has required Dave to start baby proofing around the kitchen to keep Eli out of the areas she needs to leave alone. She of course is fascinated by the process of putting the safety hook on, so has tested every lock out immediately after it has been placed on, and fortunately they are sturdy enough to handle the wrath of Eli (at least for the moment).

I'm looking forward to another great day, and if I can keep up the energy without relying so much on steroids, that would be great. I know I said this last time, but it is really amazing, if I can feel physically good throughout this for the most part, it is great. I will continue to pack on the pounds as best as I can and enjoy eating multiple meals while I can. Today is the day that the mouth sores should really be up and running, so I'm hoping some of my preventative techniques that I learned last time are able to work this time. I look forward to a night of good sleep, maybe even straight to 6 a.m.

AUGUST 15, 2013
HITTING ROCK BOTTOM IS A GOOD THING

Today my white blood cells (WBCs) officially bottomed out and reached nadir again. This is the first time it had hit nadir during this round of treatment. We are thrilled. The hospitalist actually told me that she has never seen a 0.0 before. I had actually learned about my WBC numbers when I went for my walk. I had already done my exercise in the room and was ready for my power walk on the floor to say hi to all my people, I guess by now I want to call them my hospital friends! I saw the oncologist, and she pointed out that it would be best for me to stay in my room today since my numbers were so low. It is actually okay. I really do love how big and light my room is, it is easy to hang in here, and I can always do my extra exercises in the room. I also have a new mask that I can wear to walk the halls as my numbers start to recover. The great thing about the numbers being completely depleted is this means as new bone marrow and WBCs begin to replenish there is a completely clean slate. The challenge now is making sure that these new cells that produce are not leukemic cells. This is something that we won't know until after the next bone marrow biopsy which ideally will be the first week in September.

This was Dave's first day back at work since this whole ordeal began. I certainly noticed a difference on my end since he is back at work. I didn't get my daily visit from him on his own today, which was usually a few hours in the middle of the day. I did get to have a visit from him and the kiddos in the evening after they had dinner. It was fun, Alyssa brought some balloons which turned out to be great fun for her, and Eli. Alyssa also did a great version of her own new musical that she is putting together. I love her energy, even though the kids could only be here for an hour it was great to get to hang out and play with them. It also meant that Dave and I got to see each other for a whole hour today too.

I still feel really good energy wise today, but certainly notice that I'm calmer today now that the steroids are done. It also meant that I could sleep in until 5 a.m. instead of being up at 3 a.m. like I have been the past couple mornings.

Okay, so it is almost the weekend. I'm ready for everyone's weekend plans. I look forward to hearing what everyone is going to be up to. I know in the Bay Area it is supposed to be in the mid-nineties. I will enjoy my 74-degree set climate-controlled area in the hospital but look forward to hearing everyone's weekend plans.

AUGUST 16, 2013
MOVING ON UP

Today was another day of confinement in my room; it really has not been as bad as it could be. Since the room is long, I can skip up and down the room, and seem to feel I can still get exercise even though I can't leave. I know this sounds funny and I guess it is, but I have to get some exercise. Picture this. Here I am skipping up and down the room. I did find myself pacing in front of the window for a moment and felt like a caged animal at the zoo. I remember the jaguar just going up and down along the cage looking out at the viewers. Well, that is me walking along the window for my exercise. Even with that, I've really not felt confined at all. Hopefully I don't become agoraphobic after this experience.

My WBCs are at .1 today so are making their upward move. My platelets were pretty low, but not low enough to need a transfusion; we are thinking tomorrow I will probably need new platelets. I continue to feel good and keep finding projects or things to keep me busy. Earlier this week, the chaplain had brought to my attention another young woman who is in the hospital for a while like me will be celebrating her 2nd wedding anniversary tomorrow. She and her family were trying to figure out how they could do an anniversary celebration while in the hospital. She too is neutropenic so she can't have flowers, fresh fruit, fresh vegetables, etc., and is going through all of the chemo side effects. I realized that I had a Martha Stewart kit to make a bouquet of crepe paper flowers that I'd always wanted to make, but never had the time. Dave brought the kit to me in the hospital, and I started working on it on Tuesday. Well apparently, even though it was a kit with everything ready to go, it was still too advanced for me. Each flower was made up of 20 petals that I had to cut out, fold, and attach individually. I had the intention to make her a dozen flowers and then realized it was too difficult so I only made her 2 roses to represent the anniversary, and after starting the test rose, I decided that 1 paper flower would be just fine. It is the intention that counts right? I worked on it for most of the day on Tuesday, and Thursday and finally finished it this morning. The chaplain delivered it to the other patient, and apparently, she was very touched by it. It was nice to feel like I could do something to make someone else's day.

I forget that while I'm in the hospital for a long time, I'm not the only person with this diagnosis or who is here for a long time. Since we are all in isolation, there are rarely opportunities to meet others unless you happen to run into them in the hallways. With my last visit I wasn't ready to really meet others going through this journey, but I think I am ready now, and when I can get out of my room, I look forward to meeting this other patient, until then we will be emailing pen pals from a few rooms away from each other.

The kids and Dave came by for their evening visit, and we enjoyed an hour or so of chaos and fun. Eli learned that the soiled linens cart that is on wheels that she previously has used to help her walk on, also makes for a fun ride. Alyssa and Dave were pushing her on the cart. The kids seem to think the hospital is like a playground for them. Alyssa made me more beautiful pieces of artwork for my walls. This was the kids first week with their new babysitter and it seems like things have gone great. Alyssa is doing numbers and craft projects galore, and Eli seems to be very happy. It is nice to have things falling into place so nicely. One of the many challenges of this whole situation is how unpredictable everything is. I am a planner; I like to always be 10 steps ahead. With cancer and relying on my health minute by minute, I feel like things are so out of control. It makes it hard to plan or figure out next steps. Someone pointed out that although I speak about the kids, I have not updated anyone on Brady the dog and how he is doing. Brady seems to be adapting well to things; he has made many new friends and is enjoying his 2 walks a day from all of his new friends. People have been volunteering to walk him 2 times a day, and he is loving it. It has been so helpful for Dave and the kids to not have to walk Brady on top of everything else, so it is a win-win. We are so appreciative to everyone walking him. I think Brady probably has renewed energy, always looking forward to the arrival of his friends.

AUGUST 17, 2013
TRENDING UPWARDS

My white blood cells continue to do their thing and grow day by day. They are currently at .2, I know it doesn't sound like much but remember 2 days ago we were at 0, so any upwards progress is great. My hemoglobin is staying steady, which is also what we want. My platelets seem to be hovering just above the transfusion level.

My sleep schedule is still all funky. For some reason I was up from 3 a.m. - 5 a.m. I've always been such a good sleeper it is weird to be up in the middle of the night and not able to go back to sleep. Hopefully it will help me plow through my book faster. I was able to leave my room today, although not for anything too crazy, but a welcome walk around the third floor was appreciated. Once I get tomorrow's WBCs back, I will know if I can spend more time out in the halls walking around and out of my room. My energy continues to be good; I do get lethargic throughout the day and take naps if I need to, but again, overall I'm up and about for most of the day.

Today I got to spend a lot of time with Alyssa. We did craft projects; I taught Alyssa to do finger knitting, and she made a Neapolitan colored scarf. Then she came back in the afternoon and stayed with me while Dave ran errands with Eli. Alyssa and I just watched a movie and cuddled (I tried to close my eyes, but she was adamant that I stay awake); it was so nice being with her even if she was bossy! I'm still so impressed with how maturely Alyssa has been handling everything, and love that even though we only get little spurts of time together, it is valuable quality time. I know this is a short update; apparently my middle of the night insomnia is catching up to me. Nine o'clock bedtime here I come.

AUGUST 18, 2013
CONTINUING TO LOOK GOOD

I continue to have odd nights, I wake up for a few hours in the middle of the night and am wide awake, and usually hungry. I find it funny that I don't do much all day yet manage to maintain a strong appetite, even through the night. In some ways I kind of like these early morning wake ups. All day long hospital staff are walking through the door checking vitals, asking questions, etc. In the middle of the night, no one is interrupting me. They do have to check my vitals once, but otherwise there is this nice quiet, and I can read, email, or do whatever and not be interrupted. Today was another day of more of the same. My WBCs are holding at .2 and my platelets hit 7,000. This is the lowest I have ever had my platelets. They used to always transfuse me at 20,000, so I was surprised that I still had good energy today with my platelets so low.

The kids came by for 2 separate visits today. For the morning visit we went over to the family area (yes, I'm allowed in the general population for short amounts of time with my spicy mask on). Alyssa and I played a fun game of tag while Eli tried to run along with us and join in as best as she could. We also got to do some crafts. My walls are getting more and more decorated with all of the kids' fun projects. I started to have the very beginning inklings of a potential sinus infection today. We are watching it very closely to make sure it doesn't get worse or that I don't have a fever and trying everything to not have to deal with antibiotics. Over the last month I have had so many antibiotics I don't want to put more into my body. Fingers crossed it is just a little pressure, or maybe discomfort from too much smiling (this would be the ideal diagnosis). I had my platelet transfusion this afternoon, and it is amazing how much energy I get from new platelets. As soon as the platelets were done, I had a ton of extra energy and did my third floor rounds; it felt really good to be on the move outside of the room.

The kids came back in the evening and had dinner with me, which was nice. We got to have pizza from the place across the street. I know I keep mentioning it, but it really is fantastic. It has east coast style pizza that Dave approves of. He is very picky about his pizza so if Dave approves of this it must be good. It is so convenient, and both kids loved it for dinner.

This will be the kids' second week with their babysitter, and Dave's first full week back at work. We continue to try our new routines to find out what works best for all of us. I love that I still get to see the family; I truly believe they are a huge reason why I feel so good and am able to power through this so well.

AUGUST 19, 2013
STAYING STRONG

My WBCs are holding strong at .2, they seem to be quite content here. Fortunately, this is high enough that I'm allowed out in public for at least my walks. I had a good amount of energy this morning and did my power walk throughout the third floor only to return to my room to find out that my hemoglobin is at 7.5. I have standing orders to have a blood transfusion at 8, so of course once I learned how low my numbers were, I was then overcome with exhaustion. I wonder if I would have had more energy if I hadn't learned my numbers were low. I was able to enjoy much of the rest of the day filled with new projects, hopefully I'm more successful than I was with the paper flower.

Eli had a potentially runny nose today, so we decided to forgo an in-person visit and instead have the kids visit over FaceTime. We already do breakfast every morning over FaceTime, and tonight we did a quick dinner FaceTime. I'm sure this is much easier for Dave too. I don't know how he goes into the hospital every day. Obviously, I look forward to the kids' visit, but I know that the sooner my counts recover, the quicker I can be back home with the munchkins full time. I will accept missing one day with them not visiting, if it means I get to go home sooner and see them in person.

My potential sinus infection has not increased at all, so I'm optimistic that we were able to get on top of it early. I'm trying steam and Sudafed so hopefully to avoid antibiotics.

Remember the woman I talked about a couple days ago? She was in the hospital with leukemia and was also stuck in her room? It was her 2-year anniversary, and I made her a paper rose? Well, we were both healthy enough that we were able to meet in person in the family waiting room. It was incredible to meet another stranger who was going through cancer at the same time as me. I met her husband and her mother. We were able to share our journey and how we were handling this alone and now together. I look forward to connecting with her more. I have been researching places outside of the hospital where I can begin to meet other people who I can relate to. They have gone through cancer or are currently dealing with it. Cancers are so unique, and no one understands it if they haven't had to deal with it. I know there are great resources once I get out of the hospital that I hope to take advantage of as soon as I get home, but for now it would be nice if there was something on the third floor that I could take advantage of.

AUGUST 20, 2013
HOVERING NICE AND LOW APPARENTLY

I have decided that the middle of the night is a great time to be wide awake. I was up from 1:30 a.m. until 5 a.m. Because of that I have purposely tried not to rest today (other than a quick 30-minute nap) so hopefully I can get past this new need to be up all night long. I continue to feel really good during the days and spend the day waiting and encouraging (yes, I talk to my WBCs) my numbers to bump up. You've heard about manifesting what you want right? Well, that is what I'm going for here. I'm manifesting increased WBC numbers. Today my WBCs were at .1 which is apparently nothing to worry about, and it is expected that the WBCs will continue to hover for a while before they pick up. I'll assume that they are taking a little extra time to make fully formed non-leukemic cells, so I'll give them some extra time to create perfection. Even after yesterday's blood transfusion my hemoglobin is now at an okay level. However, I did need platelets and may require blood again tomorrow.

I still have not heard any further update about whether or not my brother is a definite match. Over the weekend Dave had a great idea and said, "Why don't you just call Stanford and get the status from them?" (He's pretty smart, it's one of the many reasons I keep him around). Sure, enough I called Stanford yesterday and heard back from them today. Unfortunately, they didn't have any further information for me, but I do have an appointment with the transplant doctor at Stanford for September 6, so we will learn much more then and should know if Ben is a definite match by then. I asked the on-call oncologist about the matching, and he said that it takes a long time, and we would not know for another couple weeks. Don't they know about my obsessive need to plan and figure out the next step?!

Although spending a month and a half in the hospital is certainly not something that I have ever wanted to do, it has been survivable. Thank goodness I have been very happy overall with the staff and the care I've been receiving at Kaiser Walnut Creek. I have a handful of nurses that I consider friends, and I truly feel like the nurses genuinely care about me and my well-being. Every day I get tons of visits from different hospital personnel with different roles all wanting to know different information from me about my experiences etc. Overall, I play nice, but on my last visit here, I was asked to provide feedback about any concerns I had, and being one who is not afraid to speak my mind and share my opinions, I was happy to pipe right up. One thing that I had been concerned about was that every nurse that did the morning blood draw did it slightly differently. Some created a sterile environment and were organized with everything neat and ready. Others would just lay things out on my blankets and leave caps in my bed etc. at the end of the blood draw. One even got blood on my PJs. Now if I just wore the hospital gown, this wouldn't be a big deal, but these were my personal pajamas. I shared my experience and how it would be nice if it how they set up and cleaned up from drawing blood was more consistent. I noticed right away upon my readmission this time that now every nurse does the blood draw the same. They all create a sterile environment etc. I appreciated seeing that not only did they ask for feedback and listen to it, but they even implemented it. Now that I know they follow through, I'll get my list ready of other bits of feedback. I bet they regret that they asked me for my opinion.

Of course, a good day wouldn't be complete without the kids' updates. Alyssa had a great day and got to hang out with me at the hospital for most of the day. It was so fun; we colored and even did some preschool numbers and letters. She really enjoys spending time at the hospital and it is so nice that she and I could hang together. I am so lucky that afterwards my mom was able to take her back home. Meanwhile, Eli got to enjoy only child time with the babysitter, so it was fun for everyone. Both kids came by for a quick and more chaotic than usual visit in the evening. They really know their way around the room. Eli starts at the fridge where she pulls out her juice of choice and then she goes to the kid's activity closet and starts to pull out all of the possible toys that she might be interested in playing with. I know I only get a short time with the kids each day and it is really fun, but I find after their visit I am exhausted. I have just enough energy to sanitize my room and do my clean up routine after they leave. As soon as I say goodbye and close the door, I immediately pull out the Clorox wipes and wipe down everything they touched while they were here. I am not generally a clean and tidy person, but I want to keep this space as tidy and germ free as possible. I hope I can keep these habits going when I get home.

AUGUST 21, 2013
50 NIGHTS IN THE HOSPITAL

Tonight is my 50th night in the hospital. I know I got 3 nights at home in between my two stays, but I can't believe I've been in the hospital this long. I had a better night of sleep last night, I was awake many times, but I was always able to go back to sleep. I woke up with a pounding headache at 3 a.m., and unfortunately it continued throughout the whole day. Even with pain meds it never fully went away. I think that it might be sinus related, so we are continuing to monitor it, and they started me on an antibiotic for the sinus infection. Grrr… I did not want to get back on antibiotics. I also got a very low-grade fever in the evening. I took it very easy today and will continue to do so and nap frequently until I'm back to myself. My WBCs are still at .2 and since I had the headache, they encouraged me to stay in my room today. Fortunately, it was another beautiful day, so I was able to enjoy the view from my room.

I had a meeting with the RN Leader of the oncology floor in the morning and discussed with her my idea of offering patients a chance to meet each other, share experiences and know someone else going through something similar. She thought it was a great idea, and she wanted to present it to her team. They actually had a meeting scheduled for this afternoon where they would discuss things that they can do to better patient care and how they can continue to offer the best to the oncology patients, so I had impeccable timing to bring it up. I am hopeful that this idea/program can get off the ground, and I may even be able to get it implemented before I leave. Not only could patients meet each other, but we could play cards, do puzzles, etc. We are all here, and most of us are just dealing with the waiting game, so we have time on our hands. For me, not only do I like the idea of getting together, but being able to lead and follow through with a project gives me a sense of purpose. Yes, I know my goal here is to stay alive, and believe me I am working on that. In addition, I want to feel like there is something I can do, help build a program, know I am giving back.

I learned that there were some other patients who had heard about me, and one older woman who brings a lounge chair with her when she is here. She had apparently offered to let me borrow her chair while she goes home. Unfortunately, that message never got passed on to me, but it was so nice that she wanted to share with me. It is funny when I move in and out of my rooms, Dave wheels in my mini fridge on a dolly. We each have things that help us survive our long stays here.

Today was very low key, and I'm hoping to get rid of this headache tonight. Dave and the kids weren't able to visit this afternoon, but I was still able to do FaceTime with them which is second best.

Okay, I'm looking for game apps; they don't necessarily have to be free if they are good. I'm already playing Sudoku, Free Cell, and video poker, but I would like something more stimulating that I can play and won't get bored with quickly. I welcome your suggestions.

AUGUST 23, 2013
SLIGHT SET BACKS

My fever picked up overnight, but fortunately other than the off and on fever all day, I felt much better today than yesterday. I still have a frustrating headache, but it is much more manageable. I find that as long as I'm distracted, the headache doesn't bother me; it is when I get bored it really hurts. Fortunately, I can sleep through the headache, so there was lots of sleeping today.

They continued my IV antibiotics, so I'm hoping this will reduce the fever and the headache over time. Although I would prefer to not have a fever, last time I got the fever right after I was told I could come home early, I'm under the impression that I'm just getting the fever out of the way so it doesn't surprise me at the end when I am ready to go home. I know that is an odd way to think, but it works for me so I will go with it.

My WBCs were .2 again today, so that combined with the fever/potential infection I was asked to stay in my room. I'm hoping tomorrow I can at least get out for a little bit. Today overall was very quiet, which is what I needed.

Dave and the kids came in the evening, and Alyssa did a rousing performance of "There are animals in my cobbler," an original number that I think is bound for the Tonys. The song was approximately 5-10 minutes long, and Eli was able to participate by following Alyssa around as she did her singing and acting out. I also got a ton of new art projects on my walls from the kids. I definitely have one of the more colorfully decorated walls here at Kaiser.

Since it is Friday, I'm ready to hear everyone's weekend plans. Bring them on. What are you up to this weekend?

AUGUST 23, 2013
GUESS WHAT I CAN EAT NOW?

Today I had a huge realization. Being neutropenic, I have not been able to have any uncooked vegetables or fruits. The few fruits that I have been eating have been canned/processed fruits and I've been drinking the juice boxes they provide at the hospital. For some reason, it took me until today to ask if I could drink packaged juices from the store as long as it is pasteurized. After talking to the nurses, doctors, and finally the dietician I was told that I can drink any juice that is pasteurized. This opens up pretty much anything, including smoothie drinks like Odwalla's. I cannot believe that it took me until today to ask, but I am thrilled. I will now be having delicious healthy fruit and vegetable juices instead of the sugar-filled fake juice boxes they give us here. Bring on all of the delicious, pasteurized smoothies.

My WBCs continue to hold steady at .2. They seem to like that number, though I would really appreciate it if they would pick up a bit; I don't think they will consider letting me go home until it is at least 2.0 so I have a long way to go. My headache was still present today but not bad at all. I realized that although something is going on because I have a fever. I found that today when I wore my new mask, it was really hurting me, and I realized the mask is tight on my head and also presses on my sinuses. I was thinking it would be pretty ridiculous if the headaches I've had for a couple days were caused by the mask that I've been wearing to protect myself. The only time that my headache was really bad was when I would stand up quickly. I'm hoping that the antibiotics kick in and it stops bugging me. I've found that no painkillers work, and last night ice was the best treatment option for me, and I actually had one of my better nights of sleep overall, which was fantastic.

I got to enjoy one-on-one time with Alyssa this morning for a few hours. We had so much fun doing art projects, some preschool prep, and even some cuddle time. She and I had a great time, and it worked out well because Eli had a runny nose, so they weren't able to come back in the evening. Poor Eli, I think she is just getting new teeth, but it is not worth the risk, and it is so tough to have her visit and not be able to play with or touch her. Hopefully we will know it is teeth for sure, and I can see her tomorrow. Fortunately, we still do a lot of FaceTime, which is also helpful because over FaceTime she can see my whole face. When the kids come into visit, I wear a mask so she can't ever see my whole face.

Okay, so my question today is geared towards the guys who shave their head and sport the bald look. Do you use anything special on your head like lotion or oil daily to keep your scalp from getting dry? Let me know your secrets!

AUGUST 24, 2013
FINALLY FREE TO ROAM

I am excited to announce that today my WBCs were .3! Yes, I finally made it to .3. The on-call oncologist told me that he, too, was excited for me but that I should be prepared and not too upset if I'm back to .2 tomorrow. Apparently with the chemo treatment that I did this time, it is common for the numbers to stay pretty low until 20-24 days from starting the chemo. I started the chemo on the 7th so we are expecting my numbers to not pick up until the 27th - 31st, but it could take longer. I had just completed a round of chemo a month before this second chemo. The best thing about my .3 is that I could leave my room today. WAHOO! I was able to not only walk the floor but also go out on the patio. I waited until the evening to go out when it was a bit cooler. It was really nice to finally get to go outside. I had a nice calm day and was happy to really have a very mild almost nonexistent headache for most of the day. I still sleep with an ice pack on my head and seem to be sleeping really well. I also didn't have to deal with my fever today, which is great.

The kids came in the afternoon, and Alyssa has started to show some of the signs of being bothered by me not being home. I think the recent change with Dave going back to work and having a babysitter during the week is a tough adjustment for her. Especially now that she realizes it is a somewhat permanent change for her. I'm hoping I get to have some one-on-one time with her tomorrow to have some more "girl time" as she calls it.

The next couple months will have a lot of changes for our family. It will be very hard, but in the long run this will be a good thing for me, my health, and ultimately our family. What does this mean? It means lots of changes.

Alyssa is always asking "Mommy, do you love me?" which is so sad to hear. She is definitely needing extra reassurance that of course we love her and lots of extra cuddles and time with her. While she was here today, we had a few minutes of time just the two of us and then had some fun playing outside. Eli got a little carried away with the flowers and decided to try to eat some of them instead of just looking at them or touching them. We will be working on that. Eli was playing peek-a-boo with my hat, and I would say "Where's Eli?" and she really seemed to be trying to say "Here I am" as she took the hat down. I love seeing that with everything that is happening they still show signs of being "normal." I know, what is "normal"? But this is something that a 15-month-old should be doing. It seems she's working on playing these games and trying to speak. I love seeing how cute they are. It really brightens my day when they come to visit.

I forgot to share my fun tip yesterday. If you ever need to get a hold of SDI (State Disability Insurance), which I hope you never need to do. However, if you do need to call them, wait until 10 minutes before they close. I have been calling them every day for the last 5 weeks at random times and every time I'm told that there are too many other people waiting to speak to someone and they hang up on me. As a fluke I called at 10 minutes before 5 p.m. on Friday and sure enough I didn't have to hold for a minute I got right through. I may try this with other government agencies that I have trouble getting through to. I'm looking forward to tomorrow and hoping to be able to continue getting out and about on the third floor!

AUGUST 25, 2013
DOUBLE TIME

The numbers are really starting to come up now. Today me WBCs were .6 which is a 100% increase from yesterday. Can you tell I'm excited? The on-call oncologist was so excited to be the first to get to show me my numbers today. He said that I was responding like a first-time chemo patient with a good solid response. He thinks that the numbers should come up quickly now, so we will both be more and more excited each day. He also is looking forward to getting me out of the hospital since the hospital is filled with so many illnesses it really is in my best interest to get home sooner rather than later. I obviously am not complaining and am continuing to cheer on my WBCs so we can get them bulked up and I can head home sooner rather than later. My primary oncologist is back tomorrow after 2 weeks of vacation so I'm looking forward to seeing him and think that he may have an update on whether my brother is a match or not. I was able to complete my exercises and add in a few trips around the third floor for the first time in a while. It felt so good to be out and walking around.

I spent a lot of time with Alyssa today. We had girl time alone together to do some crafts, eat lunch together, and do quiet time, which I really had hoped would turn into a nap for her so that I could sleep too. Instead, I kept falling asleep, and she would move or something and wake me up. It was worth a try though. I'll keep it short, fortunately everything is still moving along well, and I have really begun to realize that going home is getting closer and closer. This means the next step is right around the corner. I am continuing to try to weigh all the decisions and changes that lie ahead for us as we go down the BMT route. I hope everyone enjoyed their weekend; I know that I certainly did enjoy mine.

AUGUST 26, 2013

The WBCs continue to increase like crazy. They are actually at 7.9. If they double again, then my numbers will be too high. I never thought we would be worrying about them being too high. I stopped the Neupogen today, so we shouldn't see as big of a jump tomorrow. I'd prefer to see them stick where they are or go down slightly. I was taken off the antibiotics and had some of my other medications discontinued. This is exciting. We are reducing my meds. I was also told that as long as things continue to go well, I can go home by the end of the week. This is really getting exciting. I'm also not neutropenic right now, which means I can have a salad while I am home. I even had 2 fresh strawberries today. This is very exciting. I know that yesterday's update was really long so I will keep tonight's short. Thank you everyone for reaching out to your friends and family about places to stay. We are getting closer and closer to some good spots. We may have even found a house in Castro Valley that hopefully will work. After the 6th we will know so much more. I have my bone marrow biopsy schedule as an outpatient at the clinic on Tuesday the 3rd. We also still don't know for sure if Ben is a match, but they did say that Ben continued to be a match through the more intense matching process. They haven't yet said he is not a match, so that is a great sign. I'm sure we will get the final answer once we get to Stanford.

As usual the highlight of my day was in the evening when Dave and the kids came to visit. We got to go outside and play with a bouncy ball. Eli is still learning that she is not supposed to eat those darn flowers. She really does love the plants and waddles up to them to pick the leaves or flowers. The garden will be much more full of flowers once they discharge me! We've found, though, that the patio is the best place with the kids. Even though some poor patients' rooms look into the courtyard for the most part, I don't feel like the kids are bothering anyone with their songs, yelling, ball bouncing, flower picking, etc. Looking forward to a weekend at home so I can join in on the weekend activities.

AUGUST 27, 2013
YOU WON'T BELIEVE IT

Today was both wonderful and extremely challenging. Let's start with the really good. My blood work came back great this morning. My WBCs were 2.4; yes, they increased 300%. It was so unbelievable that my oncologist had them do another blood draw. They redid the blood draw, and my WBCs came back at 3.0. This is great news because they have increased dramatically. I really hope that the cells are whole cells and non-leukemic. We will stop the Neupogen shots tomorrow and make sure that the numbers stay strong and that I don't have any fevers or possible infections. As long as I can stay well and keep my numbers up, I should be able to go home. YEAH! WAHOO! I'm so excited! Now that going home soon is a reality, that also means that going to Stanford is a reality and is right around the corner. This is great news and is also very scary. I know I want this next step to happen, but at the same time I am also feeling scared of the unknown.

There are many great things about the BMT, but there are also some major risks that I need to make sure me and my family are ready for. Now this is all new to me, so I'm sharing this with you as I'm learning this and trying to figure out how we are going to handle it. Stanford's BMT Department provided not a pamphlet, not a folder, but a whole 3-ring binder guide about their restrictions and obligations required for their program. This requires some major changes for me and my family. One of the biggest challenges is that I still don't know for sure if my brother is a match. If he is a match, then this whole process could happen very quickly. I have a meeting at Stanford on September 6 with the social worker and then the oncologist there who will become my oncologist for the next 6 months. There is a chance that if Ben is a match they could want to start everything on the 9th of September, which means I feel like I really need to get things in place. The BMT process is 114 days long from when I start the chemo to when they let me go home. They really press the 100 days post BMT, and I have to do a chemo prior to the BMT. We live 60 miles from Stanford, which is outside of the "safe zone" that Stanford will allow me to travel during my 100 days. As a result, Stanford will not let me go home to my house throughout the 114 days (of which 35-59 are spent in the hospital). I am required to rent a house or apartment within their safe zone, which is approximately 20 miles away from Stanford. I was originally told that Kaiser provides an apartment for me, but instead they just provide a per day amount of money towards my housing. This provides us with some flexibility, so we don't have to live in Palo Alto, which is helpful for Dave's commute and for our babysitter's commute too. Oh and also Palo Alto is one of the most expensive cities in Northern California. I am sure that whatever Kaiser's per diem is, it will not cover the cost of living there.

Here's where you all come in. We are looking to rent a house or apartment in the San Leandro/Castro Valley Area from roughly mid-October to mid-December. We would prefer 2 bedrooms and somewhere where we can have the kids stay with the babysitter during the day. We are also open to the idea of a house in the Palo Alto/South Bay area but that may be outside of our price range. If you know of anything, please don't hesitate to give us a call or email. We have come to the understanding that the kids will only be able to visit me on the weekends while I'm in the hospital, which is very difficult for me, but with FaceTime I will still be able to see them every day. When I thought that I couldn't live with them for the days that I am out of the hospital, it was just too much for me. I know I can soldier through a third chemo, and everything that it entails along with the rest of the BMT, but I need to be able to see Dave and the kids everyday (as long as they are healthy) while I ride out the rest of this journey, especially if I will be at a home just resting. I truly believe that they have been instrumental in me doing so well throughout these other 2 chemos, and the joy that they bring when they visit is the best medicine out there.

The other major challenge that I'm dealing with is that Stanford requires that I have a caregiver 24/7 throughout the process. There is some confusion about whether or not I can share this caregiver with the kids, specifically at night. Can Dave be the caregiver at night for both the kids and me, or do I need to have my own caregiver? On the plus side, I've never had my own nanny. I've been a nanny but never had one. Maybe I can really take advantage of this. As I learn more about the caregiver role, it is my understanding that the main purpose of the caregiver for me is to take me to my appointments at Stanford, and help get food, do laundry, etc. Fortunately, Dave can help with the nights as well as some of the shopping and laundry, etc. I will probably need help with the appointments from other caregivers. As things progress, this will be something that we add to the Lots Of Helping Hands website on the days here and there when family can't take me to the appointments.

Just out of curiosity, is this something that people think they may be able to help with occasionally, taking me to Palo Alto for appointments? It would probably require a full day when someone signs up because an appointment that was just a blood draw for 5 minutes can turn into a 5-hour blood transfusion depending on the situation. As you can see, my mind has been busy today dealing with some actual and a lot of "what ifs." I would say throughout this process the "what ifs" are the hardest part for me, and there are a lot of them. I know that I'm the main player in this game, but in order for things to work well for me it is important to have things working well for my whole family. It was nice to get a better handle on a few things today. I had actually called Stanford and received some information directly from them about the per diem for accommodations from Kaiser and also about the caregiver. The social worker was very nice and answered my questions today that usually they answer at the meeting on September 6th. It was important to me to have an idea today so we could begin to plan and get things laid out.

After a day of thinking about this craziness, it was wonderful to have Dave and the kids visit in the evening. They just make me realize what I'm fighting this fight for, and although 100 days 3+ months sounds like a long hard time, but it is a very short time in all of our lives to have things completely disrupted so we can have fun together for a long time. Tonight, the kids were in great spirits. We played in the room for a while and were able to go outside. I'm not sure if Eli is trying to mock me since I'm not supposed to touch or be around flowers, but Eli likes to pick the flowers and shove them in her mouth. I was trying to show her that she could smell the flowers, but of course I have a mask on while showing her this, so maybe she thinks I'm telling her to eat it. Alyssa was quite excited about a new bag of chips that a nurse brought by, and she had it all laid out on the table as she slowly enjoyed her bag of chips. We also ran around the patio pretending we were butterflies, even Eli joined in!

After a long day of trying to figure things out, and plenty of tears, I fell asleep at 9ish when I started writing this, hence why it is going out at 4 a.m. This happens sometimes; don't fret that this is going out so late. It is just that I'm too tired to write and make sense at night. As always, your love and support, thoughts and prayers are all felt and so very much appreciated. Thank you.

AUGUST 28, 2013
GUESS WHERE I'M WRITING THIS FROM?

I had a rough night in my hospital bed last night; I just woke up a ton and was really restless. I think I'm just so ready to get out of the hospital. My body was letting me know it was ready to go home. The day was pretty monotonous. I did my usual laps around the floor and other exercises and felt pretty peppy for the most part. Everyone's wishes for my WBCs to chill out worked. They were down to 6.5 today, which is great. I decided in the morning that I was going to see if I could go home today. I have been off my pain meds for a while and am in no pain, I have no fever, I feel fine, and to be honest, I am a bit bored and ready to get home and hang with my family for the week and a bit before I move to Stanford.

I proposed this to my doctor. I asked him that if he discharged me today could I do my labs on Friday morning to get my blood drawn to make sure my numbers were staying strong. You are not going to believe what he said. Wait for it… he completely agreed (I'm sure it was my fierce negotiating skills). This was at 1:30 p.m., and I was home by 4 p.m. I packed up quickly, and fortunately I didn't have to meet with the pharmacist prior to being discharged because I already had all of the medications at home after my last time being discharged.

It was so fun to come home. Alyssa had known that I was going to be home tomorrow, so she was so excited to see me show up a day early. It was a fun evening just hanging out reading books and eating dinner together. Oh, and I'm not neutropenic, so I was able to have a salad with dinner and even eat strawberries for dessert. I am going to live it up these next 10 days or so while I can before I get put on a really strict diet again. It really feels so great to be home, I know I keep saying that. I'm just in disbelief. Eli was also excited that I was home and enjoyed reading books and cuddling. It's funny to watch her walk around the house where she is so comfortable and how silly she is. About 30 minutes into being home, Eli decided to slam her face into the windowsill; fortunately, she was alright and just had a bloody nose, but it did cross my mind that we may need to turn around and go right back to the hospital.

As always thank you all for your love, thoughts, and prayers. As we said at the beginning this is a marathon (and one of the only ones I plan on being a part of) hopefully we are in the home stretch over these upcoming 4 months.

AUGUST 29, 2013
LOVING LIFE AT HOME

I had a fantastic day today. It was so nice to spend time with Dave and the kids in the morning, especially when the kids jumped into bed at 6:15 p.m. and wanted to read books. I had the best of all worlds today; I was able to hang and play with the kids and then when I was tired, they went outside or to the park with their babysitter. I had a mildly unproductive day but enjoyed spending it with the kiddos and then Dave when he came home. Certainly, a fantastic first (of many) days home. Tomorrow, I plan to go to the clinic to get my blood drawn to make sure all of my numbers are still looking good. Fingers crossed they draw the blood and send me home in 5 to 10 minutes, unlike last time when I had the swollen foot and they sent me straight to the hospital. I'm actually going to even drive myself to the clinic, which will be the first time that I've driven in 2 months. I'm looking forward to a wonderful weekend at home with friends and family and just enjoying being out of the hospital. I wish everyone a wonderful weekend, and as usual look forward to hearing about what you have planned.

AUGUST 30, 2013
OUT AND ABOUT

Today I had my first successful outpatient blood draw. WAHOO!! I drove myself, which was a success, and had my results by 8:15 a.m. The results let me know that everything looked good, and I didn't need any transfusions later today. I had to wait until 8:45 a.m. for the pharmacy and member services to open up, which was a bit of a pain, but overall, it was a successful and more importantly, uneventful time at Kaiser. I even walked up the 3 flights of stairs to my car in the parking lot. I ran a couple errands, less than I had planned, but got the important ones out of the way. This may sound funny, but it was so fun to run errands. I wanted to do whatever anyone wanted or needed me to do. Why? Because I could?

This sense of freedom was something I hadn't been able to experience since the end of June. At the same time today was the first time I was out in public with my bald head and my mask. I wear a hat, but it is still pretty obvious that I have "cancer" and the face mask doesn't exactly make me fit in too well. While I was waiting at the bank to see one of the specialist people today, there were these 3 young girls probably 8 to 13 years old, and they just kept staring at me. I certainly understand why they were staring at me. I looked different. I tried to smile at them, but I'm not sure if they noticed I was smiling. I don't know what I should say. I don't want them to feel bad for looking and it actually would make me feel better to clarify why I looked this way. I welcome any ideas of how I could make me feel more comfortable in this situation. Anyway, I definitely was aware that I stood out, but overall, I was so happy to be out that I didn't really care. Since I had a pretty intense morning (intense for me) I spent the rest of the day laying low. I even slept for an hour when the kids took a nap. Isn't that fun that we all napped together?

As usual I enjoyed great fun with the kiddos and all of their energy. Alyssa put on another wonderful show that lasted about 15 minutes, and Eli toddled after her occasionally offering some harmonies. I cannot express how fantastic it is to be home. I'm looking forward to laying low over the weekend but just love that I get to do it at home.

AUGUST 31, 2013
HOME SWEET HOME!

It is amazing how much I miss some of the everyday normal activities. Today I got to pump gas and do the dishes. I'm not saying these are things that I want to do all day, every day, but the independence was so nice. I enjoyed another awesome day with the family and friends. I find my energy is picking up a bit, but I still lay pretty low compared to how I used to be. During nap time, I think I had the longest nap between the kids and me. Unfortunately, I've never been a good napper, I can't just wake up and be ready to go, I'm usually tired and dragging for ages after I nap. I am not doing any exciting exercise but realize that I really need to pick it up a bit so I am able to be as strong as possible for the next round of chemo and the BMT, which may start as early as a week from now.

I got to spend some fun time with Eli in the afternoon, which involved her grunting and getting me to unload every stuffed animal that we have in a basket over the bed. After completely emptying it, it turns out she was more interested in the basket that held everything and less interested in most of the stuffed animals. It was really fun getting back into the groove of parenting (with plenty of help) and just getting to enjoy the kids and the basic daily activities. One of my prouder moments of the night was when as a treat I let

Alyssa watch a little TV before bedtime. As you all know Alyssa is a big fan of musicals, mostly her own life musical, but she also enjoys other musicals like *Annie* and has performed as a hyena in a local class production of *The Lion King* and as I mentioned earlier this summer, she was chameleon #2 in a production of *Tangled*. In June we recorded the Tonys, and that has been one of Alyssa's favorite shows for a while. Tonight, we watched the opening number that the host Neil Patrick Harris performs. I was so proud to see that Alyssa had memorized most of the start of the opening number. Anyway, it was pretty cute to see my little drama queen in all her glory. Last night was my 3rd night at home, I'm so excited that I've already been at home longer than I was last time, feeling good, and planning on staying for the rest of the week. Looking forward to more fun and family time over the weekend and hoping that it goes by very slowly!

SEPTEMBER 1, 2013
SUNDAY FUNDAY!

Continuing to have a blast at home with the family. We enjoyed a day at the park, and I even got to check out the farmers market, mask and all. Eli got to taste all of the delicious fruit for me. I'm going big while I am home, so I even got sushi for lunch, I made sure that it was all cooked, because I don't want to take any chances, but feel that sushi is a must have since I won't be able to have it for another 4 months or more. No one napped today, which was a bit of a bummer; it is so much nicer when the kiddos take their usual afternoon nap, and I can join them. I am just so excited I don't want to miss anything while I am sleeping, and they are not. We all were a bit wiped this afternoon and took it pretty easy.

We enjoyed a cool FaceTime call from my brother and his fiancée who had hiked above Yosemite Falls and showed us a great view of Half Dome and Yosemite overall. It was the second-best thing to being able to be there camping with them. My grandma, who is 104, also got to see him and his view and was a bit surprised that he was talking on the computer live from Yosemite. It was pretty cool to see her smile and reaction. It was also difficult to explain Face-Time to someone who is 104. She will be doing this more when I'm at Stanford. I continued to pack for Stanford this morning. I go on

September 6th for my BMT appointment and am expecting them to ask me to be admitted on September 9, but they could ask me to be admitted on Saturday, September 7. I know I've told you I'm a planner. Now you can see that I'm an anxious planner. I want to be ready for anything.

I didn't think much of it as I continued to unpack and repack, but it clearly is affecting Alyssa. She started acting up, and after a time out, it became clear that she is nervous about this next step and knowing that I am going back to the hospital soon. It is interesting; we are all scared and showing it in different ways. I am sure that I am showing it by needing to be in control with all that I am packing. I've pulled out all of my suitcases. She shows it by acting up. Alyssa has really had to grow up these last 2 months, and I hope she doesn't have to grow up too much more.

I have learned nothing is definite with leukemia, and everything can change in an instant. I am really hoping that this is my last hospital stay and that the transplant is able to work with my brother being the donor (if he is a match) and that I have as easy of a time with the transplant and the 3rd round of chemo, as I have had with the last 2 rounds. I feel that this transplant will move things along in a positive direction and give me the permanent remission I need. I do realize that there are risks involved, but the outcome outweighs the risk. More important, I'm looking forward to another family day tomorrow, and continue to enjoy everyone's company. Maybe there will even be a nap!

SEPTEMBER 2, 2013

Fun family times on a Monday! The great days with the family continue. I'm really enjoying good company, and again I find I continue to really see great things in some of life's little things. I know I continue to say the same thing, but that is because it really is remarkable to realize all that I have.

Alyssa has her routine of showing off her pumping on the swings on a daily basis and also her new love of jumping and how high she can jump. Eli, too, wants to jump but hasn't figured out how to actually get airborne. She goes through the motions of jumping but doesn't actually leave the ground. She too is pretty proud of herself when she starts to do what she thinks is jumping.

Our big drama of the weekend was that after my epic day on Friday and my first day of driving I somehow managed to let the battery drain on the car. I'm still not sure how I did it? I might have left a light on. Whatever. Maybe this is a sign that I shouldn't be driving the car. We realized this yesterday but decided not to do anything about it until today. I got the car jumped, and then Alyssa and I went on a nice drive to keep the battery charged. She was fascinated by the pink sunset and the nice clouds. I love that she can remind me to appreciate the little things in life. We also watched people speed by us and 1 person get pulled over. As long as it was not us who got pulled over, it was all good. I guess I taught Alyssa not to speed. Actually, if I hadn't been driving slowly to kill time to help the battery charge it very well could have been me that was driving too fast.

I'm looking forward to a busy but fun week ahead. For local people, Mt. Diablo Mothers Club has put together 2 great fundraisers for our family this coming month. On Wednesday, September 4 (Yes, this Wednesday) when it is supposed to be 91 degrees in Walnut Creek, Yogurt Station will be having a fundraiser for the whole day. I will be there with the kids and would love to see people if they are available. Also on Thursday, September 19, if you are wondering what you are going to eat that day, there is another fundraiser at Rocco's Pizzeria in Walnut Creek. Rocco's will donate a generous portion of the total food and drink sales.

SEPTEMBER 3, 2013
BONE MARROW BIOPSY DAY

Today was the big day; I went into the clinic for my bone marrow biopsy and aspiration. This is the 3rd one that I have had in 3 months, and I have to say I do not look forward to these. Fortunately, my doctor had an easier time getting the bone marrow out of my bone this time. Last time he wasn't able to get much, and we weren't sure if they were going to be able to have enough to get the counts they needed. Even though my body is producing new bone marrow, there is not a lot since I keep wiping it out with the chemo. After performing the aspiration, they do the actual biopsy. Normally this part is slightly uncomfortable with a lot of pressure; today I would say it was on the more painful side. Normally there is just 1 biopsy done, today I got to have not 1, not 2 biopsies, but 5… yes 5… uncomfortable biopsies. They normally just perform the biopsy from one side of my iliac crest. This time since they were having such a hard time being successful from the right side they had to do the biopsy on the left side too. This means they had to do the complete procedure from cleaning the area, numbing it, and breaking through the bone to perform the bone marrow biopsy on the left side. I am glad they were able to get what they needed. Unfortunately for me this means that instead of just one side of my back being sore, now it means that my whole back will be for the next couple days. As much as I don't like it, I have to keep reminding myself that this is to help learn what the next steps will be and the pain is temporary.

Of the 5 biopsies that they got today, the first did not pull out the bone, the third pulled out bone, but the bone appeared to have a lot of cartilage and not the marrow that they need, and the 5th, lucky number 5, got a good piece of bone that thankfully was full of marrow. I was certainly less than pleased (to be put it mildly) that we had to do 5 biopsies to get a good sample, but it was better to do it all now then to go home, be sore during recovery and then find out I have to come back in a few days to do it again. Normally afterwards it feels like a bad bruise on the back of my hip. After the procedure I had last month, the pain was much more significant, and I had trouble moving from a sitting to standing position or getting up out of bed. At the moment I feel like I have a bad bruise, and I hope that the recovery goes well and doesn't affect my sleep too much. I will tell you more tomorrow. Painkillers do help reduce the pain also! I should get preliminary results by the end of the week. There is a lot riding on the results of this biopsy and aspiration.

When my WBCs started to increase rapidly last week apparently there were some blast cells present in the blood count. This is not a good thing and is usually a sign that leukemia is still around. There are still 5% blast cells in my blood at the moment (you should have 0% blast cells in your blood). They are telling me that the blast cells are different from the leukemic blast cells that I had after my first round of chemo, but it cannot be determined if they are leukemic until the results from today's procedure come back. Are you confused about this? Because I certainly am.

I am less emotional about this news than I was last month. Maybe I have become numb to this or maybe it is because I know that regardless of the outcome the next step will be the same. Don't get me wrong, I would be ecstatic to hear that I am in remission, and I continue to hold onto hope that that is what I will hear when I get the results later this week. Something that keeps me optimistic about the results is that my WBCs are looking great. They are at 7.3 today, my platelets are in normal range, and my hemoglobin has been staying consistent at 8.5 for over a week now. I am not sure if this is still left over from the Neupogen I received over a week ago, or if my body is actually recovering and keeping my numbers up, but it means I can eat what I want and be out and about.

The rest of the day went well, in the evening we did a nice walk to the park and downtown. I continue to make the most of my time at home and am also very aware that come Friday I will learn when I will be back in the hospital. I'm very torn on this. I would love more time at home right now, and at the same time I would like to get things moving forward so we can get through this next phase. You would think that by now I would have learned that I have little to no control over what happens, but NO. I want to take control of this process. Instead, I will just go with the flow and see what the BMT team at Stanford has lined up for me.

SEPTEMBER 4, 2013
ANOTHER GREAT DAY!

Today was much less eventful than yesterday but a wonderful day, nonetheless. I kept myself busy with errands, playing with the kids, and taking it easy. It was very fun to attend the frozen yogurt fundraiser and get to see friends who I've not seen in a while and meet new friends who have supported me over the past 2 months. I had not yet had the pleasure of meeting them. It is so fun to get to put faces to names, and also see such wonderful people come out in support of me and our family. I am beyond grateful for my expanding village. As I have said many times, we are so appreciative of everything that has been done for us; we truly realize how lucky we are to have such wonderful people from around the world in our lives.

It was great for Alyssa to get to be out there playing with other kids and having a great time. Eli did enjoy seeing some friends her age, though she mostly just toddled around the area and of course had some of everyone's frozen yogurt.

No news yet on the results from yesterday's aspiration and biopsy; I will certainly update everyone as soon as I have more information. Hope everyone's weeks are going well.

SEPTEMBER 5, 2013
MORE ERRANDS

Seriously I enjoy this! Another great day at home. I continue to get as many errands done as possible and enjoy as much independence as I can. I took the other car to fill it up, and one of the Costco gas guys came up to me and said that if I ever want them to pump my gas for me, I just have to honk when I pull up and they will pump my gas. I let him know that I was enjoying my independence at the moment but that I would certainly take him up on it in the future. This was great that he offered this and also reminded me that I stood out. I was working too hard to feel like I fit in, and clearly I did not.

After that experience, I was going to try something that would help make me look like I had hair again. A month ago a friend got me this cool thing that I think is technically called a Halo, but I call it bangs. It is a headband with fake hair bangs that you put under a hat, and it looks like you have hair. It's cute. Anyway, the bangs were a bit long and a bit heavy, so I made an appointment with my hairdresser (yes, I realize that I am bald and shouldn't need a hairdresser) to go in and get my fake bangs trimmed. It was pretty funny, and she was a trooper, and I now have really cute bangs again as long as I wear my hat.

I have not heard any updates from my oncologist about the biopsy results. I was so spoiled in the hospital because I would hear back quickly. This whole waiting more than a few hours for results is so odd to me. I am going to take it as a good sign that I've not heard anything yet.

Tomorrow is a really big day for all of us. We are going to Stanford for the BMT appointment. The whole family (not including the kids) are going including Dave, my parents, Ben, and his fiancée. The appointment consists of 2 separate appointments, one first with the social worker that I will be assigned to and another appointment with the doctor there who will be my oncologist for the next 6 months at Stanford. Some of the big items that we will find out are:

1. If Ben is a match as a donor, I may hear some preliminary results of from my latest aspiration and biopsy.
2. When I will be admitted to Stanford to begin the BMT process.
3. And of course answers to a million other smaller questions that we have.

I am assuming Ben is a match or else they wouldn't bring him, but who knows. I have to say that would be quite disappointing if we went through this and they tell me he isn't a match. We will deal with that if we have to.

Tomorrow will be a very emotionally challenging day, and also will offer a lot of answers to questions that we have had, so I am optimistic that I will leave with a better sense of how we are moving forward, and when this process will begin. This will be the first time that I have an agreed upon date to go into the hospital, my 2 other admissions were both unplanned and canceled since I had to go back into Kaiser, so I am curious how I will react to knowing the date that I will be admitted. I will share much more information and updates with everyone tomorrow night after we learn more.

SEPTEMBER 6, 2013
THE BIG DAY

Today was the big day. It started with me going to Kaiser at 7:30 a.m. to get my blood drawn and then we made our way to Stanford after picking up the rest of the crew. It is funny how even though Kaiser and Stanford work together for this transplant, they are still very particular about who does what tests. Since I am a rule follower, I will do whatever they tell me to do. Right now, Kaiser is in charge; I wonder if that will change after today.

We encountered lots of traffic, oh San Francisco Bay Area, even though it should have been lighter on a Friday. Now I understand why they don't want us living farther than 20 miles away from the university for the first 100 days after the transplant.

The day was long but went very well. We met with the social worker and were able to get a better handle on all of the questions we have. Fortunately, we had read the 123-page binder that Stanford wants us to read to prepare for the BMT. Fortunately, the binder is available online, so we were pretty aware of what the overall process entails. It was very interesting to be there in person. I was able to see many people who were coming for their post-transplant appointments. I need to not be scared by this and realize that in the near future this will be me. The only thing I can compare it too are the intense HEPA filter mask that you see on a firefighter or a fumigator. When they go into buildings with extreme smells. The main difference here is that everyone was bald or had a wig or hat on. They had 2 bands over the top of their head and around their neck. These hold in place the front part of the contraption. On the front of their face there was a gray rubber/plastic mask that covered their nose and mouth. On either side of the gray mask were bright pink circle filters. I assume this is to keep germs from coming in. Although most people had the original pink filter, some people had decorated their filters with different cloth designs. Local sports teams' flowers or other cotton patterns to make the overall mask look less scary. In my opinion, it was so bizarre I don't think anything could really make it look better. I can't believe that I will be looking like them once I start this process. Here I felt bad that people were looking at me with the mask I wear when I'm walking out and about now. They will definitely be staring at me once I start wearing that.

I'm sure they notice my bald head and hat. They must be realizing I am there for a consultation and will soon be looking like them. Although I am not looking forward to sporting that look. I want to get through this. I know people say, "Take it one day at a time," but I'm ready to get this over with. I know what has to happen, so let's get this done. I want to be coming into this office as an outpatient who has been successful with my transplant and ready to move on. When I get my mask, I will be sure to take a picture of it and share it when I get my own.

We got checked in and were told it would be awhile before the doctor could meet with us, so we went out for a nice lunch at the hospital. Whoever says a nice lunch at the hospital? But it didn't taste bad for hospital food. Then it was time for our 1 p.m. meeting with the oncologist Dr. M. To say this meeting was a bit intense is a massive understatement. The initial good news was that Dr. M let us know that Ben is a match. WAHOO! YES, can you see me jumping up and down. I have been taken over by a huge sense of gratitude and relief. I had really assumed that he would always be a match but to hear it directly from my doctor was great. Not to think negatively, but I had never known how to handle things if Ben wasn't my match, I won't even go there since it was not the case. Back to the good news. Ben is a match so now we can discuss the realistic next steps. Dr. M discussed all of the possible options including BMT, Stem cell transplant (SCT), as well as whether or not this is something I should do. Meaning, should I keep with the chemo I had done and then do conditioning monthly chemo for 6 months. I didn't know this last option was even an option and I had already wrapped my head around the idea that I was gonna have a BMT or SCT, so I really relied on Dr. M's expertise.

While Dr. M was determining how best to move forward, we got a call from Kaiser with the great news that we had been wanting to hear. Based on the preliminary results from my bone marrow biopsy, it appears that I am in REMISSION; this is what we have been waiting to hear since July 1. This is fantastic and puts me in a great position to have a successful BMT. Dr. M set me up for an urgent BMT. I think the reason he wanted it to be ASAP is because I had achieved remission and they wanted me to stay there before my BMT. This is very exciting and means that there is a chance for permanent remission. But this is also very scary. Dr. M laid them all out which was definitely difficult to hear, but the benefits outweigh the negatives. The plan is that I will get my brother's bone marrow or stem cells. and my body will produce his non-leukemic bone marrow, and I will be cancer free and healthy and all will be great. Wahoo what a great story right?

I wish it was that simple so maybe if I keep thinking about it that easily it will go smoothly. That is what I am hoping will happen for me. However, there is only a 78% two-year survival rate of people who have allogeneic transplants. Learning that was hard to hear, I again had to really remember why I am doing this. Dr. M said that since I was so young and overall healthy, oh yah there is that disease of cancer that is killing me but other than that I am very healthy. He is very optimistic that I am a great patient for BMT or SCT. With that survival rate things looked very promising. The other issues that he told me I had to prepare for is a common side effect called Graft Versus Host Disease or GVHD. This is when the donor or graft cells attack the recipient or host. This is very common and occurs in 40-50% of BMT patients. I'm going to let everything that I learned and experienced sink in.

The meeting was so successful that at the end of it they drew 14 vials of blood from Ben. The results of these labs will ensure that he was still healthy and ready to donate. I understand why they keep testing my blood, but do they seriously need to keep testing my brother's blood? I guess that now that he was definitely going to donate, they wanted to make sure they tested everything. I am so grateful that he was happy to help.

On the way home we received an email from the nurse coordinator setting things up for me to be admitted to the hospital on Monday the 23rd. I don't know why I had originally thought it could be September 7th or 9th, but this secure date is both wonderful and scary. I can't believe it, I get a few more weeks at home where I will be able to spend more time with my family and friends. I can run errands and help around the house. During this time I will have many appointments at Stanford and Kaiser to prep for the transplant. I really need to take it all in before I am away from the house for 3 months. WOW, 100 days in a row away from the house. I am having a hard time accepting that.

You all know what I am up to. I want to know what you are up to this weekend?

SEPTEMBER 7, 2013
ENJOYING MY CONTINUED FREEDOM

Last night I was so exhausted when I posted that I completely forgot to start by thanking everyone for all of your love, support, prayers, and thoughts throughout this process. I know we still have a long road ahead of us. We know that we would not have made it this far as smoothly as we have without all that you have done for us to this point.

It was so fun to share all of the good news with everyone, especially since it is about time we had some happy news to share. I enjoyed taking advantage of my extended freedom today by going with Dave and the kids to a local kids play area called Fairy Land. The kids got to go while I was in the hospital, but I hadn't been for a while. It was so fun to get to go with them. We watched a puppet show and enjoyed the rides for the kids. This is the first time Eli has been there since she could walk, and she was able to have a whole new view of the place, toddling through the mazes and climbing on things. We enjoyed a picnic at Lake Merritt (the lake right next to Fairyland in Oakland) and an evening swim for Dave and the kids with great company in a friend's pool. Due to the Gershong catheter that I still have in my chest, I can't go in the water. It was fun to hang out and watch them from the side. Unfortunately, the kids didn't seem to appreciate that Dave and I were ready for a nap today, and they either didn't nap (in the case of Alyssa) or took a very short nap leaving us with little down time. It's a catch for me because I know I have 3+ weeks to rest once I'm in the hospital, but I also want to get my body as strong as I can in the coming weeks to make sure I go into this transplant as strong as I can.

Apparently after the transplant I will be extremely exhausted. I will have to recreate my whole lymphatic system (immune system). An interesting analogy that the doctor made was that when a woman is 9 weeks pregnant the baby begins developing their lymphatic system and it continues to develop until the baby is born at ~40 weeks. That means that it is expected that it will take me a minimum of 31 weeks post-transplant for my lymphatic system to be near its prime. Therefore, I will be severely immunosuppressed for at least that amount of time. In my opinion, that is a very long time.

It was over 100 degrees today, so we are enjoying a cooler evening, and with all of the activity today, I am sure I will be asleep by 9 p.m. again tonight.

One interesting thing about all the chemo I was on is that I don't have any temperature control for my body. I've always run cold, but in 80+ degree weather I will still wear a sweatshirt while everyone else is in shorts and tank tops. It makes it hard to find a comfortable temperature for the whole family in the car or house, but overall, I find it more interesting than bothersome.

I hope everyone is enjoying their weekend and not too hot, or too cold for my friends in the Southern Hemisphere!

SEPTEMBER 8, 2013
SUNDAY IN THE PARK!

I will keep today's update short since at 8 p.m., it is again almost past my bedtime, darn the no napping. Had another great day; we enjoyed going to the park, going to a birthday party, and of course watching football, some good, some not so good! I really love how great I feel, so I have been making sure to get a good walk in and really try to keep up my strength. I'm eating like crazy and gaining at least a pound a week. One of the big side effects of the next round of chemo and the transplant is mouth sores and people have a lot of issues eating, so I want to go into this with a "healthy appetite" (like that has ever been a problem for me!).

My big mommy fail/major laugh of the day occurred this morning at the park. I took the kids to a cute park that has Eli's favorite feature: a steep slide. The platform at the top of the slide was not overly toddler friendly, so I was up there with Eli and asked Alyssa to catch her at the bottom. Just as I let go of Eli for her to go down the slide, Alyssa's friend asked her if she wanted a snack, and Alyssa turned her head. This resulted in Eli careening into Alyssa and knocking her over and landing on top of her. Fortunately, they were both fine and the wood chips provided a soft-landing spot for everyone. I have to admit, it was like something out of Funniest Home

Videos, and as I type this I am laughing as I think about it. Alyssa thought it was pretty funny afterwards also, and Eli was excited to go down the slide again. I am sure we will have less dramatic park adventures over the next couple weeks.

I have a week ahead of appointments for the kids and myself at both Kaiser and Stanford as I continue to prep for the transplant. I wish everyone a wonderful week ahead, and as always, keep sending me notes about everything that you are up to.

SEPTEMBER 9, 2013
APPOINTMENT FILLED MONDAY

These days are getting busier and busier. Today we carpooled as a family to Dave's work this morning because we had to take one car into the shop. Our little Honda Insight has decided to stop providing AC, and in this 102-degree weather we needed to get it fixed before it isn't covered under the warranty anymore (in 120 miles). Yesterday afternoon a fire started on Mt. Diablo, the mountain near our house. The fire is a safe distance away, but we can easily see the fire at night, and as we drove Dave to work, we were driving towards the flames and smoke, I have to say I didn't feel overly safe dropping him off with no car and a fire appearing to be much closer than it was. Fortunately, I know his coworkers can take him with them if they were evacuated.

The reason I kept the good car is because I had to take the kids to the doctor this morning for their shots. Also, Eli's belated 15-month checkup. Why do you ask did she not get her 15-month checkup and vaccinations? Oh yeah, that is right our family had a few other things going on this summer. They also have to get their MMR and polio vaccines a few months earlier than scheduled because those are live vaccines. Once I have the transplant, no one around me, including me, can get live vaccines, unless I want to be separated from them for a week after they get the shot. I feel I have been separated from them enough, so if I can avoid any unnecessary separations that would be preferred. Fortunately for Alyssa she didn't need a shot for a while, but poor Eli needed to get the polio vaccine as well as 3 other shots. Thank goodness she is a trooper, and other than Alyssa rubbing it into Eli's face that she didn't need any shots, the whole appointment went smoothly. This afternoon I continued to have a video appointment with my Kaiser doctor, where he confirmed that not just the preliminary results, but the final results show that I am in remission. This is the great news I have been waiting for since early August. Does this mean that I got an A on my test?

SEPTEMBER 10, 2013
SAME OLD, SAME OLD

I'm loving it! Another day of errands and appointments. I continue to get my twice a week blood draw (my numbers continue to look great). I also got an X-ray, and an echocardiogram to prep for the transplant. They want to look at my chest to see my lungs before transplant. Same thing with my heart. They want to make sure they are strong and also use them as starting points to be able to see if they are affected after the transplant. I have a few more appointments throughout the week that I need to get done prior to the transplant. I like that I can do most if not all of these locally through Kaiser, so I don't need to drive all the way to Stanford. I know it is only 60 miles away, but in the Bay Area 60 miles can take a minimum of an hour and up to 3 hours to drive one direction. I will do anything I can do to avoid the drive. Avoiding that long drive was not possible today; I had to drive down to Stanford today for the BMT class. It turned out to be a 1-hour power point presentation that covered information that was included in the 123-page document that I already read online. It was okay because I was with my mom, and we found a cute café/restaurant called Tootsies right across from the hospital, where we had a delicious lunch and great time together. Leave it up to my mom to find the good food anyplace. I continue to have a voracious appetite that I must take advantage of.

We also were able to check out the hotel that we will be residing in during my days in the "safe zone." Oh yes did I tell you I/we found a place to stay? After freaking out, calling hotels in the "safe zone," trying to find a house on Craigslist that the whole family, the dog, and my mom could stay in during those 100 days. We finally found a great Hampton Suites that will be perfect for us. I've heard of them but never stayed in them. It is on the right side of the bridge for Dave to be able to go to work daily and our nanny to come to easily also. You may have noticed that it is called suites, so that means that we can have 2 bedrooms and 2 bathrooms. Yes, the kids can have their own room to make a mess of themselves. There is also a middle kitchen/living area where the kids can play and we can hang out in. Can you imagine anything better? It is basically an apartment. I am very hopeful that we will be able to make it our home for a couple months.

One of the reasons we need a kitchen is that I cannot have any food that is not provided by my caregiver. In many ways that sounds great. Like I have my own chef. What that really means is no takeout food, because there could be contamination. There are so many restrictions. The restrictions include: I can't eat raw fruits or vegetables; I have to have everything cooked, and I can't cook anything myself. The list goes on and on. Some great things about Homewood Suites are that they have a washer-dryer on our floor and wait for it, wait for it. They have breakfast every morning as well as dinner and a happy hour every week night. Could it get any better? Now I'm bummed that I will not be able to eat or drink any of that, but it will be great for Dave, the kids, our nanny, my mom, anyone who visits, and other caregivers. Don't tell the hotel that we are inviting others to partake in their food. The per diem that Kaiser provides doesn't fully cover the cost of the hotel, but it covers most of it, and this is the best option we have found, so we are going for it. The other tricky thing is that we don't know exactly when we will be moving in and when we will be leaving. This is difficult with any rental but more flexible with a hotel. I'm hoping to be really friendly with them, and maybe even play the cancer card to get a little flexibility from them. Wish me luck. I am so excited to keep you updated when we move in.

Everything is falling into place, which is great.

The local fire that I previously mentioned is getting more and more contained each day, and it helps that the overall temperature has cooled off quite a bit today. Fortunately, the fire is definitely not a threat to us and hasn't affected any homes. It is still scary! Over the next few days/week and a bit, I will mostly be focusing on getting appointments out of the way. Don't worry if there is not a nightly update; I am thinking to spare you from some of the minutiae of my day. I may take a night or two off here and there from posting on the website. Wishing everyone a wonderful week!

SEPTEMBER 12, 2013
ENJOYING THE SIMPLE THINGS

The appointments keep coming. Yesterday I went to the dentist because that is something else I won't be able to do for a year post transplant. I also went to get a Pulmonary Functions Test. This was quite interesting. The test wanted to see my lung capacity, and I did a bunch of breath holding, taking breaths in, and then they also tested it after giving me a bronchodilator (inhaler). This required that I sit in an enclosed plastic booth while breathing in and out. I felt like I was on a game show. I kept hoping that money would start flying around me.

After the appointment I had an hour and a bit of extra time and took that time to look for Alyssa's Halloween costume. Alyssa has decided that we should be a family of Smurfs for Halloween. Fortunately, there was a Walmart across the freeway from Kaiser, and I was able to successfully find bright blue leggings and a matching top for Alyssa and a blue top for Eli. Dave will either be Papa Smurf, or Gargamel. I am still trying to figure out which Smurf I will be with my HEPA filter mask on, possibly Hazmat Smurf or Allergy Smurf. I will have to find one with a better ring to it. I welcome any suggestions you have. As I walked into Walmart, I thought of the more recent Facebook viral video going around showing the people of Walmart. Well today I was one of the people at Walmart, and I may make it on the next video. Here I am with my bald head (I did have a cute hat on) and my yellow medical face mask running around Walmart looking for bright blue clothes for my kids.

My second appointment was to see a dermatologist to get a baseline before the transplant. Apparently, the immune suppressing medications will make me more susceptible to skin cancer. This was a doctor that I have never met before, and I have to say I would be happy to see him again. He was young—well my age isn't that young—cute and friendly. My reaction to him may be different than his impression of me. As I mentioned, this was for a full body skin checkup, so you know what that means. If you don't, I will explain. I had to fully expose myself while he looked at every inch of my skin to make sure I had no moles or other areas of concern. Usually, I make someone take me out to dinner before we get this far, but this was part of the appointment. He did find a mole on my back that he wanted me to keep a watchful eye on, or he could remove it. To avoid needing to obsess on it, I had it removed. I know that he was probably on the more cautious side of things, but he told me no more flip-flops (this is my go-to shoe) outside, and I need to invest in SPF50 clothing. Sounds like I will be in the shade a lot and dressed in full coverage clothing year round. No more nude sunbathing for me.

SEPTEMBER 15, 2013
FOOD, GLORIOUS FOOD

We've had a great weekend; we've been keeping busy getting out and about and I continue to enjoy the simple things. I'm obsessed with food right now. I find that I am ravenous and need to eat everything in sight. I have gained 10 pounds in the last month and a bit. Isn't that crazy. Gaining 10 pounds in a month. Normally I would find this appalling, but I am perfectly content with it. Bring on the delicious food. We did a great job exhausting the kids. We knew we had succeeded because both kids took naps at the same time both days this weekend. That is a major success for us. I also introduced Alyssa to Pippi Long Stocking, or as she calls her, Pippi Lawn Stopping. I have to say even though it has been 20+ years since I last saw her, I am still a fan. We spent the evening taking advantage of Eli's ability to answer "ya" to anything you say to her. It started with, Eli, do you like having Brussel sprouts for dinner? And she quickly answered "ya." We continued to say many things we wanted her to answer, from current events to do you want this for dinner. It made things very easy knowing she would always be answering "ya." I could get used to this.

I am hoping that this week is long and productive. I say long because I really need to take advantage of this and soak it all in. I have more appointments at Stanford on Thursday and Friday before I get admitted on Monday. Although I am nervous about this next phase, I am ready to get it started, and even more ready to get through it. I am all packed, and ready to move into the hospital for a month.

Since I have experience living in the hospital, I am making sure I have everything I think I will need. I won't be bringing in my refrigerator this time but will make sure I have plenty to keep me dressed and entertained. I have one extremely large and one carryon size suitcase, as well as a backpack. I know this sounds extreme, but I will be there for a long time. I also need to put things together for the family and I to be living in the hotel for a couple months after my hospital time. You are probably thinking, *Mara, why are you worrying about the hotel stuff? Dave can do it.* I agree and I am sure Dave can do it all, but I am a control freak and with so much out of my control I want to handle all of this. Also, isn't Dave doing more than enough taking care of the kids, the house, his work and worrying about me? The least I can do is help put things together before I leave.

I also know that since Stanford is so far away, I won't have family visiting me in the hospital as frequently, so I won't be able to get my laundry done. Therefore, I definitely need to pack the necessities like undergarments and then shirts and pants enough for at least a week. Beyond clothes, I need things to keep me entertained. I can only watch so much TV; I am packing word games, sudoku, a book or two and art supplies. They say I will be too tired to do anything, but I disagree. I don't want to just lay there.

Meanwhile things continue to go strong locally. The Rocco's Fundraiser is on Thursday in Walnut Creek for anyone looking to grab a bite anytime during the day or night on Thursday in the Bay Area. Due to my Thursday appointments at Stanford, it seems unlikely that I will be able to make it out for the fundraiser, but I will try; it really all depends on rush hour traffic. For those of you who can't make it but still want to know how they can help, blood donations to your local blood bank are always welcome. Although you cannot donate directly to me, any donations added to the blood bank will inadvertently help me. It is expected that I will have as few as 10-20 transfusions throughout this transplant process and could need as many as 250 (This is obviously on the extremely high side, but I was warned that this is a possibility). Wishing everyone a wonderful week!

SEPTEMBER 17, 2013
PARKS, FORTS, AND FAMILY FUN

This week has seemed very normal. Our babysitter came down with some type of illness over the weekend and will not be able to watch the kids this week. This gives me a chance to try being a stay-at-home mom for a few days. It also makes me realize that although this week it was easy for me to step in, over the next 3 months we will definitely need emergency backups. If you know anyone who would be a good backup, we would greatly appreciate it. We have many unknowns in these upcoming months and will need to have backups for both the kids and me as we start to plan out my caregivers.

Yesterday I had an appointment in the afternoon so my brother, who not only donates stem cells and saves my life, but also babysits, came over to watch the kids. I came home from my appointment to Ben playing the guitar, Alyssa rocking out on the play drum, and Eli staring up at Ben and singing along with her signature "Ya" (with a little prompting) at the right spots in the song.

This morning my mom watched the kids for a little bit so I could go get my blood drawn. Upon arriving home from today's appointment, Alyssa and my mom had made an awesome fort in the backyard. I love seeing that the kids are all doing fine throughout all of this. That helps me feel like everything is going to be okay.

It has been fun to go to the park, do art projects, and try to keep up with the two kids and the endless mess that they leave in their path. Needless to say, that by the time Dave gets home, the dishes are piled up in the sink, and the house is a disaster. Alyssa has been sleeping in a fort in her room and has been all about new sleeping creations. She asked if she could sleep in her outside fort tonight. Knowing that she is quite particular about going to sleep. Dave and I agreed that we would let her sleep in her outdoor fort. Well, sure enough, she is out there fast asleep, and it is going to be a cold night. We will bring her in before we go to sleep. What I love about that girl is that, in typical Alyssa fashion, when she sets her mind set to something, she makes sure it happens.

SEPTEMBER 19, 2013
WHAT A DAY

Had a good morning with the kids then off to Stanford to sign consent forms. There are so many forms. It is a bit daunting to hear all of the potential side effects of the medications. Most of the meeting was a repeat of the document they provided and made me sign. I basically signed my life away, really this is life or death. I signed that by doing this SCT, I could die. I could live cancer free, so it is worth it. Scary but worth it. In addition, I agreed to be part of 4 separate studies, including 3 that will be national to help provide information to other potential patients down the road. As strange as it sounds, it makes me feel like I am doing something good and means there is a reason for all of this. If I can help with these studies to learn how to help people see what treatments work, then I am honored to be part of this.

I was supposed to attend a class at 3:30 p.m. about the central line and how to care for it, but my mom and I asked the nurse if it was necessary for us. I didn't want to be snotty, but I'd already had a central line for a couple months, so I know how to take care of it. She said the class is offered every other week. This meant that we could get on the road at 2:45 p.m. to head home instead of 5:30 p.m. I'm glad we stepped out of our comfort zone and asked. It also makes us wonder if we even needed to drive all of the way down to Stanford today. Being the rule follower that I am, I followed the rules but am bummed I did today. We went to get on the Dumbarton bridge (the main bridge to get home), and we got stuck in gridlock traffic. After an hour we made it to the light only to see that the bridge was closed (this must have just happened because it wasn't on the radio yet or on the online traffic report). Needless to say, it took us 3 and a half hours to get home from Stanford, which is only 60 miles away. It was all worth it though because we went straight to Rocco's for a great fundraiser that a bunch of you set up. It was wonderful to be greeted by so many of our local friends, new and old. I continue to be amazed by what incredible people we have in our life. I am constantly reminded via email and was so lucky to get to have a sendoff tonight. Thank you to everyone local who was able to come out tonight and support us.

SEPTEMBER 22, 2013
STANFORD, HERE I COME...

I know it has been a few days since I last posted, but I tried to stay offline a bit this weekend. We met with Dr. M at Stanford (You will hear me talk about him a lot in the future) on Friday, where he again gave me a very realistic view of the side effects and risks associated with the chemo and the transplant. After that terrifying appointment, we decided it would be nice to get out of town one last time before my transplant.

We again ventured to beautiful Carmel and made the most of it. We enjoyed walking on the beach, spending time with family. Dave and I were spoiled with a chance to even check out a movie, *The Butler*. I also probably got more exercise this weekend than I've had in a while, due to Alyssa's dislike of walking. I had the privilege/got to pull her in the wagon for a couple miles. I finally made her walk at least 2 blocks because they were very steep uphill. I go into the hospital tomorrow morning to have an outpatient procedure to replace my central line from a Gershong to a Hickman catheter. It is my understanding that they are pretty similar, but the Hickman Catheter has a thicker lumen (that is the tube that goes into my heart). I will be able to tell you more about it more tomorrow. It is disappointing that I have to have this procedure done, as it will be uncomfortable recovering from it. I have become very comfortable with my current catheter, and I had just begun to forget the pain of the last catheter being inserted. Remember how something hurts so much, like childbirth or breaking a bone? Then a few days or weeks later you forget how much it hurt. This is how I am. I finally got over the pain, and I'm afraid I'm going to have to go through it again. They tell me it is necessary because the new catheter will be able to better handle things if there is ever a situation where there is high pressure liquid, blood, saline, medication that would stress the lumen. After the outpatient procedure, I will be admitted to the hospital in the afternoon and start chemotherapy the following day.

I keep reminding myself how lucky I am. I was able to have so much time at home with Dave and the kids. I feel like I got to see Eli's personality grow so much, and she will be a totally different kid when I am back with her in late October. I had a long talk with Alyssa today about how I was being admitted tomorrow. She was sad that I wasn't staying home for much longer, but I explained, in kid terms, why it is so important that I go into the hospital now so I can be home forever. Even though she and Eli won't be able to visit me in person every day, they will still be able to FaceTime me.

This will be a long new challenge, but it will be worth it.

SEPTEMBER 23, 2013
TODAY IS THE DAY

After staying up late last night to finish packing, and eat multiple dinners, (I am not allowed to eat anything from midnight until after my procedure today, so I had to make sure I ate lots last night to tide me over). I got to spend a little bit of time with the kids this morning getting them ready, and then Dave and I were off to Stanford at 7 a.m. to try to avoid traffic. Of course, that is never possible in the Bay Area, but we tried. We made it in plenty of time and walked over to the ambulatory surgery center for my procedure. The appointment was at 10 a.m., but I didn't go into the procedure until 11:49 a.m. There was some down time between when I went to the pre-op area, and when people came in to ask me questions, this was rough because there were not enough distractions to keep me from thinking about going into the hospital and leaving the kids for a month. When the nurse came to give me my IV, I was crying and struggled to stop. I am ready to start this portion of the journey, but it is still going to be tough to be away from the kids and deal with the chemo, not seeing Dave and the kids in person on a daily basis and just riding out this storm. The procedure went really smoothly, and I was awake for the whole thing. This was different from last time in July where

I was asleep for the procedure. They were able to put this new line in the exact same place as my old line, so the discomfort post procedure is very minimal. Right now, it just feels like a cut that is healing. Dave met me in the recovery room with lunch, and we hung out there for an hour before we walked over to the hospital to be admitted.

It was nice and strange. I had an outpatient procedure which went smoothly, and I was able to walk out of the room when it was done. Then I went to the car and pulled out my massive suitcase and other luggage to go back to the main hospital. I'm glad I had Dave with me to comfort me and help carry everything. The only other time I packed that much was when I was going off to college. I'm sure I packed more than enough for the next month.

As we entered the hospital, we saw signs that said E1 unit. I had been told from the instructions in the massive amount of paperwork I had read that I was to go sign in and enter the E1 unit of the hospital. We walked into the E1 unit going through the closed double door as if I was ready to check into a hotel, only less inviting. We walked down the entrance way to the front desk. I'm sure the nurses at the front were holding back a laugh as they checked me in. They had checked in hundreds of patients. I'm not sure many of them came in with as much luggage as I had. The nurse welcomed me and walked me to my double room. Yes, you read that right; it was a double room, and the other person was already in there. In all of my hospital stays, and you know there have been many, I have never had to share a room. My heart immediately sank, and I was overcome with emotion. It finally hit me. I didn't want to be sick; I didn't want to have to do this transplant, and dammit. I didn't want to share this room. The tears filled my eyes and began to scroll down my cheeks. All of my emotions, the anger, sadness, and overall realization of what was happening came out. I was truly out of control in this situation. I was also showing my feelings outwardly. I could no longer hold everything inside. I was showing Dave, the nurse, and my roommate how upset, unhappy, and out of control I was with this situation.

I looked at my small twin size hospital bed with all of the same hospital necessities behind the head of the bed as I have had in my previous hospital rooms. About a foot and a half to the right side of my bed was the outer wall towards the inside of the E1 unit. My part of the room is barely big enough to fit a chair on the right side of me. On the other side of my bed was a curtain separating me from the other patient. If I reached out to the left of my bed, I could grab the curtain; that is how close it is. I'm not sure how the nurses are going to fit when they come in to take my blood pressure, temperature, draw blood, deliver meds, and more, but they have it figured out. At the end of my bed is the control panel. I really hope they don't put on the bed alarm. Beyond the end of my bed were a few feet of space where people could stand or walk beyond me to the other patient's bed. She is my roommate now, so I will call her roommate instead of patient; that sounds nicer and more comfortable to me. Beyond that empty space was the far wall of the room. On that wall hung the TV, and below it was a small closet. Yes, a SMALL closet; where am I going to put away all of my stuff? I will worry about that, later. Next to the closet is a sink for me, my roommate, and anyone who washes their hands in the room to use. There was also a computer screen and keyboard affixed to the wall for the nurses to use when working with either of us in the room.

As if that is not enough, stuffed into a tiny room there is one more thing. Wait for it... Wait for it. Why yes, a bathroom of course. There needs to be a bathroom, and since it is a shared room, of course, there is a shared bathroom. The tricky thing about a shared bathroom in a hospital setting is that they need to measure each patients daily urine output. They do this using something called a "hat." It is a plastic bowl-shaped container that attaches to the rim of the toilet and measures each patients urine output. Sorry if this is TMI. The nurses have been doing this throughout all of my other hospital stays. However I have had a private bathroom and toilet in my other hospital stays so this has not been a problem in the past. Now sharing the bathroom this means that every time I pee, I have to lift up the toilet seat, place my "hat" on the rim of the toilet then close the seat over the bowl and you know, do what I need to do.

Then when I am done, I need to call the nurse for them to measure it and take care of things from there. Oh and what if I choose the wrong hat? They do have our name on each one, but I still have so many questions and concerns. I don't know why this bothers me so much, but it does.

Now you are probably wondering, do I have to do this at night too? If you weren't concerned about that, too bad I'm going to tell you. At night they have given me a bedside commode to use so I don't fall making my way to the bathroom that is less than 10 feet away. Are you kidding me? I'm coming to terms with sharing a room. Okay, I can handle that. Share a bathroom. I can close the door and, well that has to be okay, but now I have to go to the bathroom on a commode with only a curtain separating me from my room-mate. I don't think I can do this. This wasn't in any of the manuals that I read. In no part did it say share a room and do your business in front of, or beside, a complete stranger. Even though I am completely against it, I will accept it. Now the only thing I can control is to make sure I don't have to go to the bathroom in the middle of the night. I guess not to be too graphic, but who wants to hear someone else go to the bathroom? I got so used to having a private room and everything there, I just need to breathe and accept what is going on.

You know how I talked about the small closet? Well this space was small for anyone, but then remember all of the stuff that I insisted on bringing for my stay. Well, where am I going to put all of that? I will have to figure that out. Dave was great and helped get me settled. I want to take advantage of not being attached to the IV pole, so I put away as much of my necessary stuff as I could into the closet. I really don't know what to do with everything I brought. While trying to figure all of that out, I put a picture of my beautiful family up on the closet door so I can look at them as my main view and remind me of why I am doing this. I also get to not only be interrupted by my nurses, but by my roommate's nurses too (wish me luck for a good night's sleep). Fortunately, I know that I will only be here for a few days until my WBCs drop again and then I will get a single.

My nurse for the evening came in and did the intake questions. I've done these so many times now, I think I could do my questions all by myself: How old are you? What is your date of birth? How much alcohol do you drink a day, a week? Do you take any drugs? Are you in a healthy relationship?… The list goes on and on, but those are the highlights. I answered the questions with a crackly voice trying to control my tears and not sound like I'm about to cry. It was hard to do because I was about to start balling any minute now.

I am fine with my answers to these and any other conversations I have with the nurse and other staff, but I think it is weird that my roommate has to hear it all. We share a bathroom which I'm getting used to, but these things just add up and are making me more and more uncomfortable.

I will make it work. Okay, enough ranting about that. I will move on.

SEPTEMBER 24, 2013
THE MASKED WOMAN

I started the morning with FaceTime with the kids. I didn't realize that something I took for granted in the other hospitals with the private rooms was that I could talk on the phone to the kids or anyone for that matter, whenever I wanted without worrying about bothering anyone else. Now things are different.

In order to stick to the same schedule of my morning call with the kids, I couldn't stay in the room. I'd need to find somewhere else to go. But where? Fortunately, there is a special family room in the E1 unit which I will now call E1. The family waiting room has 4 walls, one with a door on it that leads to the hallway. It has a small coffee table and a small table with chairs. I can imagine that when my family and friends come to visit, we will meet here. The room was perfect this morning for me to enjoy a call over FaceTime with Dave and the kids while they ate breakfast. I am so glad there was a door and hopefully the walls are well insulated because my kids were as loud as they are every morning. I think there is only a patient's room on one side. I hope we didn't wake them up. With all of the changes going on, it was important for me and the family to keep the morning breakfasts together consistent. We got caught up, the kids ate breakfast, sang songs, joked about what they were going to do during the day and made sure they told me everything before the nanny came, Dave had to go to work, and the nurses were ready to change shifts and needed to take my vitals and tell me the plan for the day. I ended the call and headed back to my room.

After my labs came back, they showed that we were on track to start chemo at 9 a.m. Going forward it will be administered at 10 a.m. and 4 p.m. Every twelve hours of each med for the next 3 days. For some reason that doesn't sound like too much, but when I realize that I only have 2 of 16 doses complete, it sounds like I have a lot more chemo in store for me. Since I've already been through 2 separate months of different types of chemo, the beginning of this round doesn't seem like a big deal. I've been through this before; I know how to handle chemo, even though it is different, they all seem the same to me. Three days is not a big deal.

I have had to stay in or near my bed for most of the day today because they wanted to make sure I didn't have any side effects from the chemo. They also need to draw my blood every 15 minutes for the first hour and then every hour for the first day. They then send my lab results to Fred Hutchins Cancer Center (FHCC) up in Seattle, Washington, to see if they need to adjust my chemo doses. Here's something funny. When they first told me they had to send my labs up to FHCC so frequently I was trying to figure out, how can they do that? It will take ages to take my blood, package it up, then take it to the airport, put it on a plane, get it to FHCC, and then get the results and respond to Stanford in time for my next dosage. How are they going to do it that frequently? Then I sat back for a minute (okay, like an hour) and realized, of course they don't send vials of blood up to Washington. They perform all of the lab tests here and send the results. Apparently, all of this chemo is getting to my brain. The reason they involve FHCC is they want additional expertise to make sure they are giving me enough and not too much chemo to keep me in remission and have a clean slate before the transplant and they also want to make sure they don't give me so too much that they kill me. Okay, now I get it. I appreciate they are getting more experts involved. I did sign my life away.

Speaking of drawing blood, this new Hickman Catheter is fantastic. I'm not really in pain after the procedure yesterday, and I think they can draw blood faster now. Honestly, I don't really notice a difference between the 2 catheters, but they seem to be drawing more each time and the vampires, I mean phlebotomists are quick, so I will take their word for it.

I met more staff members throughout the day and continued to get into the swing of things here. The better I know people, the better I feel. I'm not sure everyone is like that, but it is my nature to know a lot about everyone I meet. I know it may sound weird, but that is just me. The physical therapist spent a good amount of time with me today going over appropriate exercises and how much I should walk around the unit. I realized that I shouldn't have complained about how small the third floor was at Kaiser because the unit here is quite small and is only 250 feet around the whole E1 unit. That means it takes 11 laps to do half a mile, and 22 laps around the E1 unit to do the full mile. Look at my fast math. I think I might get dizzy if I do a full mile. Knowing that people will have trouble keeping track of all of those laps they have a board where you can flip a page over after each lap to keep track of your progress. I like that to help me but also to brag about how much exercise I'm doing.

As you all know, I do not enjoy being attached to the IV pole. The nurse that had me sign the paperwork on Thursday did say I would be attached 24/7 for fluids, but I assumed I would still get detached between chemo sessions, etc. Apparently, I was very wrong. Not only am I attached between chemo sessions, I am literally attached 24/7. When I took my shower today, I stayed attached to the IV pole and just shut the shower door on the lines. It was a bit odd, and more awkward than my usual showers with the chest catheter lines, but I will get better at it over time. I will have to learn to get used to and accept all of these new things.

In addition to being attached to the IV pole, I also received my fancy HEPA filter mask tonight. You know the masks I saw the out patients wearing with the big bright pink circular filters on it? Now I have my own. I will be required to wear this mask anytime I leave the room during my stay at the hospital as well as for the next 100 days after my transplant any time I leave my house or secured safe/health place. I knew this was to be expected; I was prepared. However, actually putting it on, adjusting the straps to fit me perfectly, brought on emotions I did not expect. Again, this whole situation is beginning to be real. The process has begun, and I am about to head into the unknown.

I was not going to let all of this new equipment hold me back. I had to take advantage of the fact that my numbers are still high enough that I was able to walk outside of the unit today into the general hospital. I received many stares. I couldn't be mad; a couple weeks ago I was doing the same thing. I get it. I look different, shoot, I look bizarre. Who wouldn't stare at this? Two little kids wouldn't take their eyes off of me and pointed. One little boy asked his father what it was. In my voice that is now muffled and sounds like Darth Vader I said it was a mask to help protect me. I don't know if it helped him, but it helped me feel better. I definitely need all of your help to come up with some good responses, because I certainly stand out in a crowd. I am also thinking of some slogans for T-shirts to minimize the horror of the mask or at least make it entertaining.

I haven't had a chance to see what this hospital consists of, so I walked all 3 floors of the Stanford adult hospital. It was fun to explore and see more of what is around. I went up to the security guard at Stanford Children's hospital; the two hospitals are connected. They wouldn't let me past them. I don't understand why. Here I was this masked woman with a huge HEPA filter mask on holding onto an IV pole. I wouldn't let me through either. I will wait to explore that area until the kids come to visit. I will do this walk over the next couple days, or until they limit my freedom and tell me I have to stay on the unit. Again, the more strength I can have going into the transplant, the better.

I was able to FaceTime again with the kids at dinner. It is always fun and chaotic to talk to the kids over FaceTime. Alyssa did a show for me, and Eli joined in a little bit. I am so lucky to have this technology to get to see the kiddos. They are so used to it that other than not being able to hug them, it is just like seeing me in person. The other night Alyssa said that she would prefer if we all Face-Timed around the table instead of being there in person. I will try to not take offense to that.

I am looking forward to a good night of sleep. Last night we had a lot of people coming into the room to check on my roommate, and I was up for the day at 5:50 a.m. as usual. I am a bit tired tonight and hope to sleep well. Tonight, the nurses will be coming in for me at 4 a.m. for one of my doses of chemo, so I will be the one causing the disturbances tonight. See all the excitement you are missing out on? Don't worry, I will keep you updated!

SEPTEMBER 25, 2013
BREAKING THE RULES

I felt really good today. I had a good night of sleep other than being up for a while after the 4 a.m. chemo. It really took me a while to get back to sleep. Adjusting to this new schedule and sharing a room is really bugging me. I had to eat a sandwich at 4 a.m. because I was soooo hungry. One thing I am loving about Stanford is the food. I know, who raves about hospital food? But here I am raving about their food. Not only is the food good, but you can also have it anytime you want it. Isn't that exciting? Here I was awake at 4 a.m. and all I had to do was look at the menu and order anything off of the menu and it arrived 30-45 minutes later. How fantastic is that? Here I was being woken up for chemo, so I figured I might as well get something to eat. Who is the annoying roommate now?

I went back to sleep for a bit and then got to do my usual FaceTime with the kids for breakfast. They are such goofballs and treat Face-Time as if I was there in person, which means they are acting wild. Thank goodness they stay put in their seats. Well, Eli really has no choice; she is in her high chair, and Alyssa is pretty well behaved. Their craziness is why it is best we do these FaceTimes in the E1 family room. Apparently, this morning, even though I had the door shut, when I came out, the nurses said they could hear the kids and were wondering where the noise was coming from. Thank goodness we didn't say anything bad about the nurses and the hospital. It is just my loud, boisterous children!

I was able to head out of the unit and into the main hospital around noon today to enjoy some nice live jazz music. The live entertainment that the hospital provides in the public areas is great. I am only allowed to go outside of the unit when the chemo is not running and when I am not neutropenic (which gives me a few more days). I am doing everything I can while I can.

Today I broke my first Stanford rule, and not even on purpose. Dave came to visit in the afternoon, and since I can only have dairy for a few more days, I had him pick me up a milkshake. I drank the whole thing and didn't think anything of it until the nurse came in and threw it away. She told me that I can't have milkshakes, especially this one. I cannot have food made from an outside restaurant. Now, I remember that this is one of the rules, but I thought it was after my transplant. I must have missed that in the 123-page rule book. Oops, now they have me on extra surveillance, and I'm considered a rule breaker. I was surprised, as I did not even think that a milkshake was considered restaurant food (obviously I know it is, but it didn't register when I asked Dave to pick one up). Here I am 3 days in, and I already have a big X next to my name (It was a pretty delicious milkshake though). I continue to eat only hospital food and feel like I continue to gain weight like crazy. This food continues to be delicious. I have to order well before I am on a limited diet.

On top of all of the food I am eating, I am getting 6 liters of saline in my IV each day and drink another 3 liters of water/juice on my own, so I am definitely well hydrated. In case I didn't have enough saline in my body, I also started doing the mouth hygiene routine, which is washing my mouth out 6 times a day with saline to prevent mouth sores. Everyone says they will get pretty bad, so I am hoping to stay ahead of them as best as possible. Ben is on his way home from winning singles and doubles in golf croquet this week in North Carolina. Did I mention my brother is not only a national but an international croquet player? Isn't that incredible? I wonder if I will gain some of his skills after the transplant. He is going to arrive late tonight. He will arrive back in California just in time to go to the clinic tomorrow to start getting his daily Neupogen shots to prepare his body for the transplant. The reason he takes this is to increase his blood cells prior to his donation. He will get 1 shot for 4 days and then they will do the stem cell donation on Monday the 30th and possibly Tuesday the 1st if extra stem cells are needed. Now we are both on this adventure together.

To help pass the time while hanging out in this double room, I have been getting to know my roommate. This is so odd; here I am stuck in this room where we are both sick, in this cramped room where neither of us want to be, not knowing what our future holds. I/we decided we might as well get to know each other. Her name is Meredith. She is a young, single girl in her late 20s. She has long, brown hair like mine used to be, a darker complexion then mine, (doesn't everyone?) and looks healthy. Shoot, we all looked healthy until we were told we weren't. I asked her why she was here, and she said she is about to have her second SCT. Wait, a second SCT? I am shocked. A second SCT; how is that possible? I thought the whole deal is, you have one BMT or SCT and that is it. Isn't that what I have signed up for? You go through all of the chemo and treatments. You have one allogeneic SCT, you go past the 100 days, you experience all of the challenges, the bad side effects, and you then survive. Once you make it through all of that you are alive. You are alive, you are another person's DNA, and you go on with life. I knew this would be hard, but I was willing to do this. I was willing to put my family through this but only once. That is what we are going to go through. Not a second time.

She went on to tell me more about her story, what she had gone through and more. It was all a blur. I kept asking questions, but I wasn't listening. When I asked her how she was able to stay nearby, she said she had been a nanny to a family that lived close to the hospital, and they let her live with them during the 100 days. Funny, she was their nanny, and now they were her nanny. Her friends rotated caregiving for her during those first 100 days. I will have to set up something like that. I keep thinking how awful it must be to have to go through this a second time. Getting to know her and meet her friends as they drop by makes me less resentful of her having to share a room with me. I also appreciate her positive attitude and outlook on everything. Knowing she did well after her transplant gives me hope. Now knowing she is having a second transplant is a bit concerning and makes me nervous. I will focus on the positive. I will continue to remind myself that, even with all of this, I am so lucky.

With the curtain open, I got to see more of the other side of the room where she was. The side appears to be slightly bigger with a large window that looks out to a courtyard. What I can see on that side of the room is a shelf along the wall where she holds her bags and other things. She appears to have far fewer things than I do, or maybe she puts them away better than I do.

I can see that the loud sound that I hear multiple times a day is actually the medical helicopter landing on the hospital roof. From the window I can actually see where the chopper lands and takes off.

I am fantasizing about how I can put all of my necessary things on the shelf and hide my bags and suitcase underneath. When she moves out and I move over, I could see this for myself as I look out the window to the beautiful courtyard. Is it bad that I am already planning how I will take over that side of the room? I really am a nice person, but one can dream, right? My guess is she will be neutropenic and move out of the room before I can. This will let me have seniority of the room. Okay, I will get back to living in the moment. On that note, I wish you a wonderful evening. I look forward to giving you my update tomorrow.

SEPTEMBER 26, 2013
I HAD ANOTHER UNEVENTFUL DAY

As far as side effects are considered, I did find that I was slightly more lethargic than I have been and I am experiencing a bit of nausea, but my nurse was right on top of it and gave me some IV medication that helped me get rid of the nausea and made me a bit tired. I was able to FaceTime with the kiddos. However, I have to wear the masks when I am outside of my room. Since I go to the family waiting area to talk over FaceTime, I have to wear the mask until I get a single room. I am not sure how that will work. I want to go to the family room so I don't bug my roommate, but I have to wear the mask in that room. If I am wearing that mask, my speech is muffled, and it is hard for them to understand me. I will have to figure out how to make that work. Again, let this be my biggest problem. I welcome any ideas of how to solve this problem.

My numbers are still really strong and well above what they have been the last couple months prior to my being in remission. My day became a bit more special with a visit from Alyssa and my mom today. This makes up for me not being able to FaceTime with her and Eli this morning. As always, Alyssa had ideas of what she wanted to do including wanting to put on a performance only after everyone else in the hospital left the common area. We got to have a tea party, but I quickly learned that I cannot drink real tea with my mask on. I just had to pretend and got to show what a great actress I am. We also had a chance to explore the beautiful gardens in and around the hospital. It was fun exploring around. Alyssa was certainly a bit bored, but it was really great for me to see her.

I have now completed 10 of 16 rounds of Busulfan (chemo) and will have my last dose at 4 a.m. Saturday morning and then I will do 2 days of another chemo before enjoying a chemo free Monday. The chemo I am on now is going to make me lose my hair again, which is kind of sad. I hadn't mentioned that, although very short, my hair is growing in really nicely and evenly. The thought of losing my hair again is annoying. I am happy to know that I have the ability to grow my hair back. It only took about a month and a half to go from shiny bald to shaved-head look gives me something to look forward to. I had been afraid it was never going to come back or was going to come back all spotty.

Wishing everyone a wonderful Friday, and I look forward to hearing what everyone is up to this weekend.

SEPTEMBER 27, 2013
FRIDAY FUNDAY!

The nights seem to be going pretty smoothly. I get my chemo at 10 p.m. and 4 a.m., and I am able to usually sleep through most of the chemo prep and connecting, which is nice. I had a rough emotional morning though this morning. I am not sure if it is because I am nervous about what is coming ahead, or if it is because I have been confined in between 2 curtains in this room for too long without a window to look out of.

A therapist came to help me do visualization this morning. Now hear me out. I am really trying to be open to many things, but today I was not. As I was slightly sitting up in my bed, a woman came into the room. She said she was there to help me do meditation. I've never wanted to do meditation, but I said I'd try it. She sat in the chair next to my bed. Remember how I told you how little space there is between the wall and the bed? Well, the chair she sat in took up all of that space next to my bed. She was pretty much touching the bed with her legs. She told me to close my eyes and start visualizing a beach and the sand on the beach and the waves crashing on it. Blah, blah, blah. The tears came rolling down my cheeks; I could feel my chest heaving. I didn't want to think about that. I was just freaking out about what my future held. What was going to happen the next few days? I tried to be polite, but I told the woman to please stop. I couldn't keep listening to her. I think she was surprised that I interrupted her. She did stop and quickly left. I'm not sure what I expected was going to happen next, but I'd rather accept my sorrows than listen to her. I know her words and visualizations are probably very helpful for others but not me. I'm not sure why I acted that way, but I did. It could be anxiety, or it could just be me.

I don't know why I am so weepy. Maybe my emotions are just so much more on the surface. Like how I show joy when I when Alyssa visits or how I feel sad about the fact that I cannot be as mobile as I was at home, and I feel like some of my personality is lost behind the mask that I have to wear. There are so many feelings and emotions that I've never had to experience.

At the moment, when the kids visit, we have to meet in the family waiting room. Going forward, the kids will be able to visit in my single room as long as they are healthy. Tomorrow, I hope to be able to walk around the rest of the hospital with Dave, Alyssa, and Eli. I know that for the rest of the month I will need to stay on the ward and not be able to explore. When Alyssa came to visit today, she put on a great performance with some beautiful twirls. She is also having a bit of a tough time with me being back in the hospital. I know that she, like I, will be able to get through it. It is tough to watch her struggle too. I FaceTimed with Eli tonight and she is doing great, which is very nice that at such a young age she appears to not be phased by this. As the day went on, I was feeling better. I walked around the ward 22 times, completed that full mile, turning the page on the lap board over with every lap I completed. I was very proud of myself and wanted to make sure everyone else saw all that I was doing. Later in the evening, I did another half mile too. I'm pretty impressed with myself.

One of the wives of another patient told me I was an inspiration, and she was going to get her husband out walking too. Sure enough, he joined me on the next lap. In the afternoon, I had an art lesson with an art therapist, and we did a cool puzzle picture.

For the art therapy project, we had 6 people, including Alyssa, each color in a different piece of a puzzle picture that I drew of a rainbow. It was cool to see the different takes on what the rainbow could look like. I also loved that, although the puzzle could be taken apart, it could also be put back together.

My roommate will be going home later tonight, so I will be able to either move to the window side of the room or possibly get a single bed, if one is available. Since my numbers are still so good, I am not a priority to move to a single room though. At this point, I will be happy with anything other than this tight, dark area. I would love the window part of this room. I think it will be very helpful psychologically to move to the window that overlooks a beautiful garden. Now I can design the area like I had already thought of. With the amount of hospital rooms I've been in, maybe this could be a new career. Hospital room design. I will have to think about that.

Wishing everyone a wonderful weekend!

SEPTEMBER 28, 2013
SATURDAY QUICK UPDATE

I completed my 16th and final dose of busulfan overnight. I was able to get moved to the window side of the room around 10:30 p.m. last night. This is great. Now I have a view of the outside world again. It was just in time as my new roommate moved in around 11 p.m. Yes, I had 30 minutes to myself. I didn't realize how much I should have appreciated my old roommate. Overall, she was mostly quiet, and when her friends came to visit; they weren't loud at all. This new roommate is not the same. She is older and did not seem to acknowledge that she was sharing a room with me. She was on the phone a lot and would talk very loudly. Not only on a cell phone but on the room phone, and she would let it ring all day long. I hope she isn't here for long or that I get to move out soon. This makes me realize that I need to appreciate what I had. It is funny because when I share a room, part of the problem is their noise, but the other part is that I try to be a good roommate, so I am always talking quietly and trying to be kind. Apparently, not everyone feels the same. That is my new roommate. Anyway, I hope this doesn't last too long.

I had a great visit with the kids this morning. The hospital is a completely different place on the weekends. The hallways are so empty. We were able to run in the halls and we took the kids down the hall to the children's hospital. The children's hospital is attached to the other hospital, but there is a security guard separating them. Once you pass the security guard, you leave what is a gray, dull colored building into a more brightly colored orange, green, and other colored children's hospital. We found a cool model train set up in an enclosed glass area approximately 12 feet by 12 feet square. The kids could press buttons to turn on the trains inside it, and they would ride around the track. Both kids loved pushing the buttons and cheering as the Jelly Belly car came by. It went over bridges and through tunnels. Over water and through mountains. It was so fun watching the kids have so much fun. I enjoyed these moments of normalcy that I was able to experience with my family. Dave and I were able to catch up briefly while the kids had fun. The enclosed train set was so detailed with so much to see we were constantly finding more and more to explore.

In the afternoon, Dave stayed and hung out with me as I began my first of two courses of Cytoxin. Doesn't the name itself of the chemo sound dangerous? Like a toxin. Again, why am I letting them put this into my body? I had to stay in my room during this chemo because it is going to cause a decrease in blood pressure (there is a concern of lack of balance and falling) and makes me pee a lot (instead of peeing once every 2 hours, I now have to go multiples times an hour). Remember how I talked about sharing a bathroom and having to pee in a hat and calling the nurses to measure it? Well, this is now happening multiple times an hour. Also, I started to get my first real chemo side effects this afternoon too. This includes tingly mouth, headache, nausea, and restless legs (Dave actually had to transcribe this for me tonight. He really is amazing!). I am hoping to minimize these side effects tomorrow. I'm calling it an early night tonight to get some extra rest.

SEPTEMBER 29, 2013
SUNNY SUNDAY

I slept really well last night after my traumatic evening reaction to the chemo. Whatever meds they gave me not only helped my nausea and headaches, but also calmed down my restless legs. It also helped that my roommate was quieter, or if she was noisy, I slept through it.

Fortunately, today was far more successful. In the morning the kids came to visit as usual, and we went further into the children's hospital and found a fun room for the kids to run all over. I know I said this yesterday, but it really is amazing the difference in how crowded everything is during the week versus how calm and vacant the halls are on the weekends. It made it great for both kids to run around the halls and enjoy the place without us being worried they were going to get run into, get lost, or get into trouble. I am so happy Eli is walking around more because I can't imagine her crawling everywhere.

I was able to walk around a lot today until my FINAL, yes let me emphasize FINAL, IV chemo started, which made me remain in bed. Fortunately for Dave, this meant that he was able to watch a couple football games, since I wasn't forcing him to be out and about the hospital with me. Dave is also enjoying the hospital food when he comes to visit. He has helped taste some of the other meals that I haven't had a chance to try yet.

I've not talked about Ben at all recently. He has completed 4 days of Neupogen with minimal side effects. He has had to endure the bone pain that we warned him about. Thank goodness some Claritin and a little Norco are helping him with the pain. Tomorrow, he goes in for his final shot and will begin the Stem Cell Donation an hour after he receives that shot. If for some reason more stem cells are required, he will do that donation on Tuesday, and then I will receive the donation later in the day Tuesday.

My roommate was moved out this afternoon only for a new male roommate to be moved into my room. I can't believe I have not only a second roommate but a man. I mean I share a room, and a bathroom, at home with Dave, but I have chosen Dave; this guy is a complete stranger. I am not pleased about this, can you tell? Luckily, he was a temporary roommate. It was supposed to only be for 30 minutes. I decided I would be nice and put up with it, but it took 5+ hours until they moved him out.

I am going to bed!

SEPTEMBER 30, 2013
TRANSPLANT EVE

I am writing this from my new single room, which is awesome. It is so nice to be back in my own space. I think all of this complaining is really a great distraction from me freaking out about what is to come with my transplant.

Let me tell you about my new place. As you walk into my room, it is so much lighter than the previous room. The average-size window looks out onto an open space filled with, wait for it, all of the cranes and tractors that fill the construction site that is building the new hospital. You are probably wondering why am I so excited about a construction site? I am going to be in the room for quite a long time, so I am getting to watch the construction workers all day long. I'm expecting them to look like the workers from the Diet Coke commercials from the 90s. Do you remember them? If you don't, you have to look them up, and you will understand my excitement. This could be very exciting. It will definitely not be boring, and really, I will not be bothered by the noise. They have prepared me for being very tired, so noise should not be an issue.

Now that I am in this room, I know I am one step closer to transplant date. I'm nervous, excited, and mostly ready for this to happen.

I slept fantastic in my new single room (have I said that enough?). It was great to get to wake up and FaceTime with the kids without having to put on my mask and go into the family waiting room. We had a great chat this morning and Alyssa is really receptive to communicating this way. Eli also enjoys a good version of Itsy-Bitsy Spider to polish off the morning chat.

Fortunately, I am up nice and early because of the construction workers. They apparently like to start work early and don't keep it quiet for the patients. I was able to open my curtains to admire them working hard, and unfortunately unlike the Diet Coke ad, they do not stop in front of my window and drink a Diet Coke with their shirts off at lunch time. I can wish, can't I? Also, they don't look like the construction workers in the commercial. Unless they are the same actors, just 30 years older now.

Today was my day of rest and the day that Ben donated his stem cells. I know I talked a bit about how they take out my bone marrow and my bone marrow aspirations but nothing about how they take out the stem cells. Remember how Ben has been taking Neupegen for the last 4 days to increase his blood forming cells? Well, he has been producing extra blood cells, so he has plenty to donate. He went into Stanford today, sat into a chair at the clinic and they put an IV into one arm where they pulled blood out of his arm, the same way they would draw blood for a blood test. Then they take that blood from his arm, cycle it out through a machine that cycles out the stem cells. The rest of the blood is then put back through an IV in his other arm. Overall, this doesn't affect him because he is constantly producing healthy blood cells from his marrow. The whole process takes a couple hours and is done while he is awake. His donation went well, and he had enough stem cells filtered today so he doesn't have to come in tomorrow and donate more, which I know both he and I are pleased about. The medical team came in today, and when I say team, I mean 7+ medical professionals gather around my bed just like in the movies. They all told me how things are going and answered my questions to let me know things are all set for tomorrow. Apparently, the transplant will take place tomorrow afternoon because tomorrow is a busy transplant day and they go alphabetically, so Solomon is at the end. The transplant should take 30 minutes total and is transplanted through my IV, so it should be pretty anticlimactic.

If you think about it, this is pretty crazy. Here Ben has spent 4 days boosting up his blood cell count. Then he took an additional couple hour to get the stem cells cycled from him. All of this and then it takes only 30 minutes to deliver this to me. I am fascinated to keep learning about this. Today was also the last day that I can have dairy, so I made sure to order ice cream for lunch. The diet isn't too restrictive this time. But no dairy for 100 days is going to be a bit challenging for me, given my love of cheese, milk, and ice cream.

I know there have been times throughout these last few months when my time at the hospital has been compared to a spa experience. Today I had a harpist come into my room and play a few songs to me. It was pretty awesome and very relaxing.

OCTOBER 1, 2013

TRANSPLANT DAY! TRANSPLANT DAY! I AM BEING RE-BORN!

Today is my new birthday! I got new stem cells, and the new adventure begins. As usual I woke up and got to FaceTime with the kiddos. It continues to impress me how natural Alyssa is with Face-Time and how she just jumps right into the conversation as if I was there and nothing had changed. Eli is a bit more relaxed, but also feels very comfortable laughing out in response to something going on or joining in on a little sing along.

After the call, I had a visit from an RN skin specialist. There is some concern about my new central line and whether there is some infection. They drew cultures this morning for them to grow, and we should hear something back later tomorrow. I don't have any fevers, and we are all hoping it is just a reaction to the new bandage they use here. If it is an infection, they may completely change my line, so fingers crossed it is just a sensitive skin reaction to the bandage. Who knew I was so darn sensitive?

My transplant was at 1:30 p.m. in the afternoon. I got some Benadryl ahead of time to reduce my immediate allergy that I may have to the stem cells. Then they brought in the stem cells. It was both exciting and a bit anticlimactic. Here it is, a bag of stem cells that are my new life. I can't explain it. I am looking at a pale, creamy colored liquid in a small bag maybe 3 inches high, 6 inches long, and .25 inches deep that is going to give me new life. If I didn't know what was happening, I would think this was a small banana milk shake in a bag, but I digress. They hooked the stem cells up to my IV pole and started them flowing into my central line. I stared as the liquid slowly but steadily came out of the bag through the tubing into the catheter that went directly into my heart. This was my life. My new life. My brother's stem cells were my new life. As there got less and less in the bag, the nurse massaged the bag to make sure that every stem cell made it out of the bag and in to me. It took about half an hour for them to completely leave the bag and get into my body. It was weird; here my life was being saved. This small bag of cells was my brand-new life. Everything from this moment October 1, 2013, on was a brand new me. I still can't believe this has happened. After all of the cells went into my body, they kept checking on me every 15 minutes and told me to call them if there were any issues or I felt weird. The only thing that felt weird was that my brother and his cells had just saved my life. That was so surreal.

I spent the rest of the day with my whole body just feeling exhausted, but my eyes weren't tired. It was odd, even my cheeks seemed ready to rest. This is the beginning of a whole new adventure. Today is now known as Day 0, and over the next roughly 21 days, while I am in the hospital the transplanted cells will try to take over my body and produce new bone marrow. Apparently, the stem cells are smart enough to find their way into my bone marrow right away. Isn't that strange they just know where to go?

As a result, I am on immune-suppressing medications to keep my body from fighting off the new cells, and tomorrow I will take a new chemotherapy that will help suppress the new stem cells, so they don't fight off my organs as we create a happy living environment for these new cells in my body. It is expected that the cells will begin to graft around day 18 to 24 and that is when we will be able to determine if there are any GVHD issues and how well Ben's cells will take over my body.

Does this make sense to you? It is starting to make sense to me, but it is very confusing. Basically, my body's cells, my organs, my skin, and pretty much everything I was born with, including my original blood and bone marrow, is made up of one cell type. They have all worked together in one happy family. Happy until I got leukemia and my cancerous blood tried to kill me. That is why we had to do the SCT. Now as of 1:30 p.m. this afternoon, I have Ben's healthy stem cells, who have taken over and are producing new bone marrow. All future blood that is produced from my bone marrow will produce his DNA. Isn't that incredible and weird? That is why they are giving me all of these immunosuppressants and other meds to help my body create a happy environment for everyone to live together peacefully.

My 100 days post stem cell transplant count starts today.

The whole medical team came in and brought me a small cake that said "Happy Birthday" and sang the birthday song to me. I assume it was dairy free, but who cares? It was delicious. They didn't bring in a candle because there is something about fire and all of the oxygen around, but the cake was enough. I know I'm getting distracted, but wouldn't that be awful? Here you are getting a new life, and you catch on fire. That would definitely be a bummer. My re-birthday is October 1, 2013. I love birthdays, so having 2 a year to celebrate will be so fun.

Thank you everyone for celebrating today with me; hoping to have a very uneventful 100 days.

OCTOBER 2, 2013
DAY 1 COMPLETE

I am thrilled to say today was a completely uneventful day. I continue to feel good and was able to do my daily exercises and walk half a mile around the unit. I was able to take the methotrexate (the chemo being used in a low dose as an immunosuppressant) without any issues, and otherwise just rode out the day. I know it sounds boring and it kind of was. With that being said, boring is good. I haven't asked about all of the bad things that could happen, but I really don't want to know about them. I want to stay bored. I have enjoyed most of my nurses here. I really love the nurse that I had yesterday and today. She seems to approach things like I would, and I like when I present her with an ailment or a situation, she then lets me know all of the options available to me. She also likes to let me know what to expect or ideas of things that she thinks have worked for other patients. This helps me feel more prepared for the unknown. During rounds today I was sporting my brightly colored pajamas with watermelons and parrots on them while sitting on a brightly patterned blanket. The doctors told me that I was certainly the most colorful patient today. Wahoo, I love standing out in a good way. The cultures for my line have come back as negative, so it looks like I should be able to keep my line in, and don't need it replaced. I also heard a rumor that I should be moving to a new room tomorrow that has a double door, so there is never a time when the air from the hallway comes directly into my room. This will be helpful when my numbers drop, and I become neutropenic. This room may afford me a view of something other than the construction of the new hospital. We will see! Continuing to hope for non-eventful days to come!

OCTOBER 3, 2013
DAY 2 MOVING ALONG

Day 2, another successful day. I have a calendar on the wall to help me cross down the days until I get out of the hospital. Although it is not promised to go home on day 30, it is at least something to look forward to. Right now, we are playing a bit of a waiting game to observe me and make sure I don't have any chemo issues, or any GVHD symptoms. GVHD is the term that I will use going forward for any of the grafts (the donor cells) arguing with the host (my cells or everything other than my original blood). Simultaneously my numbers are finally dropping, so I should be neutropenic (have no white blood cell count) in the next day or so. Then we will wait for the new stem cells to begin producing new WBCs in the coming weeks. I was able to go out of my room again today, so I enjoyed my 11 laps around the unit. It is a bit monotonous and amazing how quickly my muscles have become weak. I am mostly sedentary and am already noticing it. Apparently, according to the housekeeping guy who cleaned my room today, I walk the unit more than any other patient he has seen. That is a bit concerning, since I only walk the unit for less than 20 minutes a day. It still makes me smile.

Alyssa came to visit this afternoon and her visit coincided with the art health specialist. We did a really fun Modge Podge art project together, and Alyssa rocked it. We had a big heart, and we got to Modge Podge different pieces of tissue paper all around it. It turned out to be beautiful. Alyssa also played her favorite game, Doctor (it is different from how she did it a Kaiser). She stands there and lectures me about all of the biopsies that she is going to have to do. My favorite line from her today was, "Well, I've never been here before and don't have a lot of experience, so let's do the transplant again on Sunday if that's okay." She didn't exactly make me confident in her abilities as my doctor.

I FaceTimed with Eli and Dave in the evening and came up with a pretty awesome magic trick. Dave or Eli would throw a tissue towards my head on the iPad, and I would put the tissue on my head, so it looked like the tissue had gone through the screen to me. I am not sure if Eli fell for it, but Dave and I thought it was pretty clever and funny. I'm looking forward to visits from the kids over the weekend.

What is everyone else up to? Wishing everyone a great Friday and weekend.

OCTOBER 4, 2013
DAY +3 GOING STRONG

I have realized that napping is not for me, so last night I went to bed before 9 p.m. and woke up for the day at 7 a.m. this morning. Unfortunately, I was woken up at least 10 times last night to either go to the bathroom, get my vitals taken, or take meds. I certainly look forward to being home or at least at the hotel, so I will not be interrupted throughout the night. I'm bummed that that won't happen for a few more weeks.

I had a very full day today. Alyssa came for a visit in the morning with my mom and stayed for the whole day. We enjoyed decorating my calendar, which charts my blood count each day. (I'm surprised this craft isn't done in preschool. Wouldn't every kid love to have a calendar charting their blood counts!?) We were also able to enjoy live music out in the main hospital. Alyssa even had a song dedicated to her. I am super lucky that my numbers are still high enough that I am allowed to go out of my room and out of the ward into the general hospital.

I had the PT come visit today and put a stationary bike in my room. It looks like the double-door room I was planning on moving to was given to someone else, so I am getting more permanently set up in my room. The stationary bike is set up with a chair behind it and I am supposed to sit in the chair and pedal the bike, so I don't accidentally fall off of the bike. Clearly the PT department knows how uncoordinated I am, and it is safest for me to use it this way. We will see if I can handle 30 minutes on the bike watching the construction.

In the late afternoon, Eli joined Alyssa, and we were able to hang in the room a bit. Eli found that after inspecting the whole room, her favorite thing was to crawl under the head of my bed when it is in the sitting position and play with the hydraulics. I don't think the nursing assistant was very impressed with my parenting skills, and she asked me to pull Eli out from under there. Eli will need to find somewhere else to play. We also got to go out and enjoy the gardens for a while in the evening. I put on my hazmat mask, and we headed on out to enjoy the beautiful Stanford hospital gardens. The kids played around, and we just sat back and relaxed, occasionally ruining the relaxing environment by yelling out to Eli and Alyssa telling them not to pick, step on the flowers, or wreak havoc on the gardens. I must be feeling okay, since I am still able to yell at my kids.

I continue to feel really good overall. I was tired today; I want to start trying to nap, but it is really hard to find a time to nap when the hospital staff is constantly walking in and out of my room. They seem to be pleased that I have not yet developed mouth sores. Other than random infections, the main thing that most people who have had a transplant deal with is mucositis, or mouth sores. This is what I am working so hard to avoid. To avoid them, I am constantly rinsing my mouth out with a mouthwash mixed with salt, water, and baking soda. They told me to do that every time I stand up. That has become a habit, and it helps me avoid getting mouth sores. I will keep doing it. I remember how sore my mouth was when I had that tongue sore last month, and I hear these could be much worse. I do not want to have to deal with that again. I'm looking forward to more time with the kids and Dave over the weekend. Have a great weekend!

OCTOBER 5, 2013
CALM QUIET SATURDAY

Things continue to go smoothly. My numbers are dropping rapidly, and I am still not neutropenic, so I am enjoying being able to leave my room. Dave and the kids came over this morning and we enjoyed checking out the model trains (our go to location) in the children's hospital. The kids love watching the train and of course running around. We were also able to go hang out in the gardens, and I enjoyed what could be my last day out in the open air. The nurses chose me to test a new bedside phone/remote control holder. I felt so honored that they had 1 holder and chose me out of all of the patients to be the one to test it out and give feedback at the end of the weekend. Apparently, they think that I may be able to offer a strong opinion (I've only been here 2 weeks and they seem to think I am opinionated; I am so surprised!). I spent the rest of the day doing art projects and watching movies. It was a pretty chill Saturday, and I've decided that I would much prefer a quiet, potentially boring day to one filled with pain and discomfort. Sorry for the short update, but it really is pretty quiet here.

OCTOBER 6, 2013
DAY 5 AND I AM NEUTROPENIC

I am officially neutropenic today. I am very glad that I spent as much time around the hospital and gardens yesterday as I did because I will spend the next week or more in my room. I am still in the room with the beautiful construction view but should be moving to a double-door room in the coming days. Hopefully it is one with views of the gardens. I spent way too much time in bed today; I really will need to find other places to sit in the room or things that I can do to keep me mobile and moving around. I did the stationary bike today and know that that will be something I struggle to do daily for 30+ minutes a day. I know you are probably wondering why I can't even do 30 minutes on the bike, but I just can't. It is boring, and I can't seem to force myself to do it. Seriously, I welcome any advice you have. I don't know why I can't make myself do it, but I just can't. Also, since my platelets have dropped so dramatically, I can't do anything that may be rough on my muscles like the tension band, etc. because it could make me bruise. Once again, I am so delicate. Hopefully I see the PT tomorrow and can work with her on things to keep me active and not lose too much muscle mass.

During rounds, the doctors let me know that things are going better than average; you hear that? Better than average! That is what I like to hear. They are very pleased with my progress. Unfortunately, I am not out of the woods; the doctors and the nurses have been mentioning the potential side effects that I need to realize I will experience to one degree or another. I am certainly very lucky because Ben was a 10 out of 10 match, and we have the same blood type. This puts me in the position to have potentially few side effects with the transplant and overall grafting.

The kids came for a quick visit with Dave around lunch. Since we have to stay in the room, it is a lot tougher to keep them entertained. Alyssa loves riding the stationary bike (possibly I should grab on to some of her enthusiasm about the bike), and Eli enjoyed walking around the room and yelling (I am sure the other patients just love hearing her scream). The kids left in the early afternoon, and Dave stayed until he got kicked out at 8 p.m.

Tomorrow is our 7-year wedding anniversary, and since he has work tomorrow, today was our day to celebrate. I have to say our hospital dinner wasn't exactly the fanciest or most romantic anniversary dinner we have had, but it was wonderful to have his company, and this anniversary certainly has more meaning than any previous anniversary. It was not how we expected to spend it. You know how many people say "in sickness and in health" in their wedding vows? Well, we thought it would be clever to say "in good times and in not so good times." Well, we certainly are trying those out. I'm glad that things are on the up and up, and I hope next year is a much better anniversary.

I have now been in the hospital for 2 weeks and expect to have 2 more weeks in the hospital before I can go to the hotel. I'm looking forward to the days flying by. I hope everyone has a fantastic week ahead.

OCTOBER 8, 2013
DAY +7 UPDATE

These last 2 days continue to go quite well. My WBCs keep dropping, which is what we want them to do. I am hoping that they bottom out soon so the numbers can start to trend upwards again. I am starting to feel a potential mouth sore forming at the base of my tongue, but it has not progressed too terribly over the last couple days. I also have one in my throat that just feels like there is a pill stuck in my throat. I also have a runny nose, so they did an uncomfortable test on me today to see if I have a cold. To test it, they stick a bristly brush up my nose until it is horribly uncomfortable and then they send it out to be tested to determine if I have a cold or not. If I was any normal person—yes, I'm not normal, have you figured that out yet?—they would just let me ride this out. Right now, they want me to tell them about any little thing going on, and they want to be hypersensitive and test it all. While we wait for the results, everyone who walks into my room has to wear both the usual mask and clear glasses so they don't catch my germs if I am actually sick. I feel pretty good overall still though, so hopefully this is all just precautionary.

I learned something very interesting today. Next year I will have to redo all of the shots that I have accumulated over the years because

I will not have any immunity. That means everything from polio to whooping cough, MMR, Hep B, chickenpox, etc. I had not fully realized that previously. Think of me like a newborn baby who is susceptible to everything out there. I guess I have to be hypersensitive and careful about everything.

The kids and Dave got their flu shots this afternoon, and Alyssa was a big girl and didn't get the nasal spray (it is a live virus, and I can't be around her for 7-10 days with it) but got the shot instead. Since I have no immune system, it is crucial that everyone around me have all of their shots and be healthy, so I am not exposed to all of the viruses. Remember the woman at Kaiser who celebrated her anniversary, and I made her the paper rose? Well, I have stayed in touch with her, and for our anniversary she sent us a throw blanket to keep me warm at the hospital. It is neat to have created a friendship as we both go through this journey. There are great people I meet at and around the hospital. I'm also loving this incredible village that you have become and are a part of.

I am hoping to have a good night's sleep tonight and feel good tomorrow. I look forward to telling you all about it tomorrow.

OCTOBER 9, 2013
DAY +8 AND DOING GREAT!

My WBCs continue to go down, which is exactly what we want. They are at .4 today, and it will be interesting to see where I bottom out this time before my new WBCs are produced. My blood dropped to 7, so I had to have yet another blood transfusion to increase my numbers. It is funny; we want some numbers to decrease and some to increase. At the end of the day, it really is a numbers game. When the medical team did their rounds, they let me know how impressed they were with how things were going for me. Apparently, days 6-9 are usually the most difficult, and with today being day 8 I have remained pretty much side effect free. I have noticed that I have some mucositis in my throat, so it feels like a mixture of having a pill stuck in my throat and a very bad sore throat. Even with the discomfort, I am still able to eat but I find that I have reduced the amount that I consume. It is funny to the medical team that what I think is an ailment they think is nothing. I will again consider this good news. I am so glad that I am not experiencing what others deal with. Every medical practitioner that walks in my room is shocked that I am still eating solids. I may be the one stem cell transplant patient who gains weight while here instead of losing it.

We found out late in the afternoon that I do not have the rhinovirus that they tested me for, so people no longer need to wear clear plastic glasses when they visit me. The glasses people were wearing were to prevent visitors and staff from droplet exposure, just in case I happened to spit in their eye while talking. It seemed a bit overkill, but better safe than sorry, I guess.

I did my usual FaceTiming with the kids at breakfast and dinner; it was pretty chaotic but nice to catch up with Alyssa mostly and listen to Eli grunt in response to any question. Eli is also fascinated with peekaboo where I cover the camera with my finger and then remove it. She thinks it is hilarious. I was able to do the exercise bike for 60 minutes today, which I thought was pretty good. After that I learned that riding the bike that long with a very low hemoglobin tired me out more than I realized, and I started dozing off around 6:30 p.m. tonight. Between the discomfort from the mucositis and my exhaustion, I pretty much was done for the night around 7 p.m. Hence why I am writing this at 12:45 a.m. Thursday morning. They told me to try to keep biking but only for two 15-minute sessions tomorrow, so I don't overdo it.

As the days go on, I get closer and closer to a potential discharge date. Realistically, it will be sometime between the 16th and 22nd of October as long as things continue to go well. I know many of you have expressed an interest in helping out as a caregiver for me over the next 3 months, and I wanted to see if you could let me know if you are still interested. The caregiver role mainly includes driving me to the clinic at Stanford and spending time with me there. It would also include making my meals (some may just need to be microwaved) because I am not allowed to handle the food uncooked or cooked by a restaurant. There may be some grocery shopping with me and just being my buddy for the day. There would potentially be lots of down time to read, etc. It would be a full day job for the day or days that you helped out. If you are interested, definitely let me know any days or date ranges that are best for you or dates that do not work. Having to ask people to be a caregiver is one of the more difficult parts for me just because I am usually so independent and accepting that I am so dependent on others is hard for me. I know you understand. Have a wonderful day.

OCTOBER 10, 2013
DAY +9 A DAY OF REST

I was definitely feeling fatigued today. Some of the fatigue is due to the medication I am taking, and other fatigue is just to be expected due to my low blood count and my body trying to get ready to build a whole new immune system. My numbers remain low, and my WBCs are still at .4. I am hoping this is my nadir, so I can only go up from here. My platelets are still low this morning but not low enough for another transfusion. Around breakfast time, I got a bloody nose that would not stop, so they decided that they had to look at more than just numbers and move forward with a transfusion. Thank goodness I couldn't leave my room today because I looked ridiculous with gauze pads stuck up my nose to stop the bleeding. I hope the bleeding stays stopped. They have given me a clamp that I can put on my nose if that happens again. If I was swimming, this might look normal, but hanging out in the hospital it is just bizarre.

Today my special visitor was an acoustic guitar player. I was about to take a nap before he came in and felt like I could move mountains after he left. He played a few pop and classical songs and really lifted my mood. How cool is this? I had my own private concert that showed up in my room. He was great; he had his idea of what he was going to play and also took requests. I forget how much I love music and how it can turn my day around. As if a private concert wasn't enough, his visit was followed by a 30-minute massage. This was really relaxing. I am not sure how I got on the list to receive a private concert and a message, but I am not complaining. I hope that I will be getting more massages throughout the rest of my time while I am inpatient.

I continue to have the pain in my throat and feeling that there is a pill stuck in my esophagus. Today they started to medicate me for this, and by the end of the day they set me up with a PCA (Patient Controlled Analgesia) which allows me to give myself the medication with the click of a button. I must have been annoying them by asking for medication constantly, but that is fine. Remember how much I love being in control? Well, here I am back in control of my medication. Basically every 20 minutes I can press a button to have more of the pain medication injected into my IV. It is kind of fun and has allowed me to minimize the pain and bring it to a tolerable level. I hope it works well throughout the night so I can get better consistent rest than I've had the last couple nights. I also like that I can do it as soon as I feel I need it and I don't have to call the nurses and wait for them to come. I don't know how much of this is really the medicine being delivered and me just thinking that there is medicine being delivered. Even if it is a placebo effect, I will take it.

The kids and I had some difficulty connecting on FaceTime tonight, so I had a conversation with Alyssa over the phone. She is so mature on the phone and really has good phone manners (I know I was surprised too). Tonight, she wanted to play operator and would talk for a few minutes, then pass the phone off to Dave, then take the phone back and pass it on to Eli, etc. It was pretty cute. I get to see Dave and the kids tomorrow night and really look forward to much needed cuddles in the future. I'm looking forward to hearing what everyone is up to this weekend. Hope fun plans are in store.

OCTOBER 11, 2013
DAY +10 AND THE WEEKEND BEGINS

I will keep this Friday night update short. I continue to have a hard time sleeping. We have upped the constant medication for tonight, and I can still press the PCA if I feel the need for additional pain medication. Last night I found myself pressing the PCA pretty frequently, and although my eyes were so tired, I could not sleep; I just laid there and cat napped all night long.

When I FaceTimed with Dave and the kids in the morning, Dave thought FT had paused, but no, I had actually fallen asleep for a second. Alyssa may have a little cough and runny nose, so we decided it was best to have the kids not come visit until we know she is okay. That is definitely a bummer, but hopefully she is feeling better quickly, and we can hang out when I get out of the hospital. Really, I know this is best for me and will help keep me healthy and able to come home as soon as possible. With that being said, I am really sad. Seeing them all in person is what is keeping me going.

Alyssa and I decided that we would do a FaceTime project so we can have virtual mommy-daughter time. I was pretty lethargic all morning, so it was probably a good thing that the kids didn't come by in person. Luckily that didn't keep me from riding my stationary bike. I kept it to 30 minutes this time, so I don't overdo it like I did last time. Again, I know this doesn't sound like a lot, but it is a good amount for me, and anything is better than just staying in the bed and doing nothing.

Today is my second day with my HGB at 8, and if I am below 8, they will give me a blood transfusion. Based on how my numbers have trended in the past, I am assuming I will need a blood transfusion tomorrow morning. As the day went on, I had the art therapist meet with me, and I was inspired to try my hand at a Matisse picture that is one of the Jazz series. I still need to finish it up. I also had another complimentary massage this afternoon. I feel pretty lucky to have all of these extra relaxing services provided to me. I wonder if I will also get a pedicure and manicure. Is it too much if I ask for one?

They say the mucositis should get better in the coming days, which makes me feel pretty lucky. I have my last dose of methotrexate tomorrow. They have to check my sodium bicarbonate levels all night because the more basic my ph levels are, the more smoothly and quickly the methotrexate will move out of my system. It is the methotrexate that is the last straw when it comes to mucositis. Ideally the methotrexate will do its job, and the mucositis will leave too. I welcome getting my 4th and final dose of it done. I'm dozing off as I write this, but my nurses just came in and said that my HGB is at 7.1 so they have to do the transfusion as soon as the blood arrives instead of waiting until tomorrow morning. Hopefully the interruptions related to that don't mess with my sleep too much.

OCTOBER 12, 2013
DAY +11 A NICE DAY FOR LOUNGING

Today was another chill day. I continue to struggle when it comes to sleeping well at night. I wake up every half hour to every hour. I also dealt with vomiting today just because I stood up. I was not dizzy, nor did I feel nauseated. I just threw up whenever I got up. Isn't that odd? I've never dealt with that before, and I hate throwing up. I did feel better throughout the day as the pain meds remained under control, and I am optimistic for a more controlled night. I was able to spend the day relaxing, and I was treated to another acoustic guitar concert today. I could really get used to this. He kept asking for requests, but then I didn't know what to request. I welcome suggestions for when he comes back. I will have to keep a list handy.

I had to turn down an offer for a complimentary massage today (Isn't that ridiculous turning down a massage? What is wrong with me?) because I was busy with all the nurses jumping in and out all day.

Meanwhile the kids went to Carmel with my parents, but they forgot the pack 'n play so Eli is sleeping quite happily in a doggy play yard. I'm not sure if that makes for a fun play yard or could be considered torture, but we will call it fun. Don't call Child Protective Services on us (CPS). Eli is loving it. It has a door that Eli can sometimes open. Regardless, she is sleeping really well, so we may just have to revisit this idea (it has to be better than having her sleep in a drawer). I am optimistic that I will be able to see the kids tomorrow, even if it is a brief visit. I am off to bed, wishing everyone a great Sunday!

OCTOBER 13, 2013
DAY +12 AND THE NUMBERS ARE MOVING UP

I am excited to say that I am continuing to make great progress. I received another blood transfusion in the middle of the night, and even though I was still up quite frequently throughout the night, I slept better and was in less pain last night than I had been the previous nights. I actually woke up 2 separate times because of an error on my part. I know I mentioned earlier in the week how I am so tired that I sometimes just fall asleep in the middle of conversation. Well, I am embarrassed to say that while I was getting a sip of water in the middle of the night, I must have forgotten to swallow the water the first time and forgot to put the glass back another time. This resulted in 2 separate occasions where I was awoken with a startle because I had spilled water on myself, either from my mouth or my cup. Isn't that ridiculous? Have you ever done that? Woken yourself up by surprise? Please don't tell me I'm the only one to do this.

I was up bright and early and made sure to get my shower in. I know I don't talk about my showers often. Don't worry, I do shower somewhat often. It continues to be such an ordeal to have to have help getting all taped up to make sure I don't get my lines wet. I guess I should be happy I don't have to worry about washing my hair and drying it and all of that. That actually used to be something that took the most time. Back when I had hair, it would take forever to wash, dry, straighten, and overall style it. Now I don't have to worry about all of that. Now it just takes forever to get my line covered up. Then the shower is pretty quick.

In the morning, I had a nice visit with Dave. We were able to hang out, play travel Scrabble, watch football, and just relax a bit. I continue to get 4 liters of saline a day and have been holding on to a lot of it, so they are going to reduce my IV liquids since I drink at least 2 liters a day of liquids anyway. I am hoping this will help me lose some of the 8 pounds of water that I have been hanging out in my body for the last week. Isn't that wild? I've gained 8 pounds, and they are saying that is all water and saline.

The kids came by in the afternoon for a quick visit. Eli seems surprised to see me in person versus over FaceTime. Alyssa and I did a fun art project, and she gave me feedback on the art I did the other day with the art specialist; it seems that she approves of the project. I love that I have been able to make the hospital a fun place and not scary for the kids. That has been one of my goals. The hospital is somewhere we have been spending a lot of time together. I want to make sure it can be a friendly place. Somewhere they look forward to visiting me and not scared of it.

In the evening, I learned that my WBCs are continuing to go up, and I am no longer neutropenic. This is so exciting. This means that the stem cells are engrafting, and I will be out of the hospital quicker than originally planned. My goal is Friday the 18th, I am hoping I will continue to meet the criteria they want me to meet so I can be discharged on time. To make sure I meet that goal, I will continue to do my 30 minutes (or more) biking in the room to increase my stamina. Clearly, I will need to stretch and walk more before I get out of the hospital! I hope they let me out of the room to do more than the pedal bike. Okay, I'm off to bed now. Here's to a better night of sleeping.

OCTOBER 14, 2013
DAY +13 IS TODAY DISCHARGE DAY?

Discharge is so close I can feel it. I've learned not to get too excited about things, but I am. It is so exciting to have my numbers continue to increase. I spent the day walking around the floor and trying to be as mobile as possible. Oh yes, they let me walk out in the hallway within the unit. I love feeling free again. I continue to wake up bright and early feeling like I have tons of energy, and then after ¼ mile of walking, I feel like I need a nap. Fortunately, today when I arrived back at the room the massage therapist had just arrived, so I was able to enjoy a nice massage and nap at the same time. I don't know if I will be able to live this spa life again. The medical team came in to go over my care plan. Since I am engraving, they feel that my few side effects should diminish quickly as my WBCs pick up. The medical team is very pleased with how things are going and are switching me to oral medications instead of IV to help me transition home. They are also taking me off of the pain medications, over the next day or so. As long as things continue on the upward trend that I am on, they expect to have me discharged by Wednesday. I asked if we could put off the discharge to Friday to better match my caregiver's availability. Doesn't this sound ridiculous? Here they want to get me out of the hospital, and I am asking for me to stay. This is crazy. I'm sure whatever needs to happen will work. I will speak with them again tomorrow and see if Thursday works for them. I was able to call the hotel and set up a room for me starting on Thursday the 17th. The day continued to fly; by early afternoon I was ready to have another nap and finish up all of my unfinished crafts.

I also noticed that my hair has been doing some funny things. I know I have mentioned that I didn't have any hair and for the most part I don't, but the hair that I do have is really strange. Although my hair has made a mass exodus, I still have portions of my eyebrows to take care of. Yes, when chemo gets rid of your hair that doesn't just mean your head hair. It means everything. Including your eyebrows, your eyelashes, your armpits, your legs and your... well, you know, everything. I'm mostly concerned about my head hair, and I will have to figure out how to cover it up. Maybe I will go back to wearing a hat. It is starting to be fall weather, so a hat will be perfect.

I enjoyed FaceTime with the kids for breakfast and dinner. Breakfast was pretty quiet, and unfortunately, I was the joke. I kept closing my eyes occasionally if the conversation didn't include me. Alyssa would suddenly yell out, "Mommy, are you paused or just asleep?" This morning many times I had to admit I was asleep. Fortunately, dinner was more productive, and we could actually converse. I got to hear all about her day and let her know how excited I am to hang out with her outside of the hospital after Thursday. I am certainly excited to get to spend more quality time with Dave and the kiddos. Eli did her occasional yelling at the screen to get my attention (yes, it works). I really am so excited that my conversations over FaceTime will soon be over. I was to hug them in person soon.

OCTOBER 15, 2013
DAY +14 MOVING ALONG

This will be a quick update. I was all ready to be discharged on Thursday. However, since I am no longer neutropenic, I got kicked out of my single room and moved into a double room with a roommate today. Grrr, not a double again. I hope this is not for too long. I did get a window, but this made me realize that I do not want to wait until Thursday, so Dave is going to pick me up tomorrow afternoon/evening. This gets me out of here sooner, and as long as nothing crazy happens tonight, that will be the plan. The doctor was very impressed with how things have gone for me, and he said if he had known things were going to go so well, then he would have had me do this as an outpatient. What, I didn't know it was possible to have a SCT as an outpatient? Why didn't they offer that to me?

After I leave the hospital, I need to come back to the infusion center daily, or every other day to keep getting my blood and certain medication levels checked. And for them to continue to monitor me over the next 85 days. The kids are very excited for me to be leaving the hospital. Alyssa was so excited, and in response to her excitement, Eli was also giddy, clapping and squealing with joy! I am ready to be with the family. There is still a long road ahead, but things have gone really well so far.

OCTOBER 18, 2013
DAY +17 ENJOYING LIFE OUT OF THE HOSPITAL

On Wednesday I spent the day anticipating my departure from the hospital. I was able to check out some live music in the main hospital, but mostly just hung out waiting for my discharge. In the evening Dave came to the hospital and sprung me. I was discharged in the evening and headed to my new home for the next couple months in Newark, California, just across the bridge from Stanford. We got there and the kids were already there; it was great to see them and actually get to hang out with them without my mask on. The hotel we are staying at provides breakfast every day and dinner Monday through Thursday, so although I cannot partake in any of that, Dave and the kids can, which is great. Dave won't have to cook for them, and everyone will get a chance to breathe on that front. A night at the hotel was much better than a night at the hospital, and at least when I woke up it was of my own accord and not because nurses were waking me up every hour. I also wasn't getting my labs drawn at 5 a.m. like I had been for the last few weeks. I do find I wake up at least once in the middle of the night to eat. This may be a new habit.

On Thursday, I went with the kids and Dave to breakfast downstairs, which was fun. The fully cooked breakfast was great for all of them. There were so many options, which was fantastic. It was a bit weird to sit there with my gas mask on while everyone was eating. It is important for me to start setting new routines. I got out of the room, took the elevator downstairs, sat for breakfast, helped the kids get breakfast, and will start this as our new routine. I love a schedule and practicing getting out more. Since we are at the hotel, it is also kind of like a vacation, right? I will tell myself that.

OCTOBER 20, 2013
DAY +19 GETTING SETTLED

Things continue to go well during my recuperation at the hotel. We had a fantastic weekend. I never mentioned that on top of all of the restrictions during my hundred days post-transplant, I also cannot drive. That meant that I need someone to drive me to my appointments at the clinic at Stanford to get my blood drawn. The area I go to is called the ITA. I don't actually know what that stands for but that is where they told me to go. When I arrived there, it was the first time since the hospital that I felt like I didn't stand out. At least half of the people in the waiting room were wearing masks and the other half were their caregivers. No one looked at me like I was a freak. They all knew what I was going through. I walked up to the counter to check in and told the woman my name with my muffled voice through the thick rubber and filters of my mask. She didn't ask me to talk louder or repeat myself. Everyone talked this way, and she knew how to hear us. It really felt good to fit in. They called me in a little bit later than my scheduled appointment, but that's okay; we had freed up our whole day. These appointments are going to be something I do a few times a week, so we will get used to it. A nurse came into the waiting room and called my name. She had a hospital wristband with my name on it and put it on me. She then took me to a big open room with 10 medical chairs. I was directed to one with enough room next to it for Dave (my fantastic caregiver today) to sit down in. There was a curtain that we could close around us to create a private environment, but I kept it open. It makes me feel claustrophobic, and there's no need for privacy now. After I sat down, I noticed that there was a wall of windows with some chairs next to it. Next time I will ask for a chair next to the window. My nurse took my vitals, and drew my blood, and asked if I had any symptoms or concerns that I wanted to report. It is funny, when they are asking for issues, I start racking my brain. Shoot, what is going on with me; do I have anything I should be telling them while I am here? What if I under report? Fortunately, all is currently going well. After 30-60 minutes I met my nurse practitioner (NP), who updated me on my blood levels. My numbers continue to increase at a slow and steady rate. In addition to the blood draw, they did a chest X-ray, which they do every other week during the 100 days. The chest X-ray is done to make sure my chest remains clear. Fortunately, I've never had any issues with my chest and lungs. I hope this stays the same way throughout these 100 days. Not to get ahead of myself, but my NP said that if things continue to move forward in as positive of a direction as they have been going, I may be able to go home sooner than expected. She also said that since things were going so smoothly, I only have to come in to the clinic 3 days a week instead of everyday like I thought I might have to. This is good in so many ways. I'm glad my body is doing so well health-wise. I'm also glad we don't have to spend a whole day driving all the way to Stanford sitting through the appointment and then driving all the way home. It takes a whole day. I would much prefer to let my body rest and heal at the hotel.

While at our appointment on Saturday, we had some friends from out of town watching the kids, and I used to babysit their two girls who are 13 and 9 now. It is so surreal to me that two girls that I used to babysit are now old enough to babysit my kids. On Sunday, we broke all of the rules. First thing in the morning Dave and I drove back to the house to grab some more things that we needed here. It was a success, and fortunately there were no emergencies. To keep the weekend fantastic, Eli and Alyssa were surprised by their Baba and Deda (Dave's dad and stepmom) with tickets to Disney on Ice. Dave went with them, which broke yet another rule, leaving me alone for 4 hours (again nothing happened, so we are doing well with successfully breaking the rules). Alyssa dressed up in her Belle dress, and both kids had a great time (I was surprised to hear that the show even held Eli's interest). When they arrived back from the show Eli was asleep in the car, so Dave sent Alyssa up in the elevator by herself. I was waiting for her and will never forget when the door opened. She was in the back corner of the elevator with her beautiful dress on, a Tinkerbell cup in one hand, a light-up toy spinning vibrantly in her other hand, and a huge smile on her face. She was so happy!

OCTOBER 21, 2013
STAYING STRONG DAY + 20

I went back to Stanford today for my appointment; this time we brought cupcakes for the staff and had even better service. We are not above bribery. The big drama is that I have an ingrown toenail, but we are just watching it to make sure nothing crazy happens. I am also having some initial signs of GVHD with some redness on my back and chest. It is actually a good sign to have minimal GVHD, which lets us know that the new cells are taking over; we just don't want it to be too dramatic. I am hoping to keep it to some light redness. I keep learning more interesting things about stem cell transplants. For example, it is important that I know all of my brother's allergies because I will now be allergic to everything that he is allergic to. Fortunately, he doesn't have too many allergies, and many of them I already had (allergic to cats and seasonal allergies), so it shouldn't be too different from what I'm used to.

Today I laid pretty low; I find I get pretty tired the day after my Stanford appointments, so I was taking it easy. I made sure to get in some walking and ran some errands but otherwise took it easy. I continue to eat really well, including at least 1 if not 2 meals in the middle of the night. I know I mentioned this before, but I may be one of the few transplant patients who gains weight during the process. I hope everyone is having a wonderful week so far.

OCTOBER 27, 2013
CONTINUING TO MAKE PROGRESS DAY +26

Things continue to go swimmingly. This week my appointments were on Wednesday and Friday, and my blood work continues to look great with my platelets at a perfect level showing the new cells are taking over. The GVHD rash is still present, but my NP says she is not impressed, which is a good sign. I really want to keep things non-impressive. I have remained so non-impressive that they are now only having me come into the ITA at the cancer center 2 times a week; this will be great. I was excited to learn that by mid-November I can start eating dairy again (I still have to wait 14 days). I have been testing out all of the soy cheeses, ice cream, and almond milk, and although they are palatable, I look forward to the real deal again. I had an awkward moment on the shuttle from the Stanford cancer center over to the parking garage. Normally we get on the bus, say hi and thank you to the driver, and keep it pretty quiet on the 5-minute shuttle ride. On Friday, there was a shuttle full of people and the driver says, "So, how is everybody doing today?" A very nice gesture, but this is a bus full of people leaving the cancer center, obviously we all could be doing a bit better. There was just silence; how do you answer that question? "Well, we are all leaving the cancer center, so we are glad to be alive?" Maybe I'm being a bit critical but seriously. What did he expect? It was very nice, though, for him to be saying hi. I will leave it at that.

The kids continue to do great; they went to Ardenwood Farm on Thursday (This is the oldest working farm in the Bay Area). Both kids climbed a huge haystack and took a horse-drawn carriage ride through the farm. I've been taking afternoon naps and woke up the other day to the sound of children screaming; sure enough it was my kids out on the sports court outside my window. They were having fun. What more can you ask for? They love the sports court and enjoy running around, trying to play tennis. Eli enjoys trying to escape through the netting behind the basketball hoop. Alyssa has asked if she can move into the hotel permanently; we will see how she feels after a few months here.

I know that the main focus through all of this is obviously to get healthy and stay alive, and with this I have so much guilt that I am putting Dave and the kids through all of this. I keep telling myself that this is helping my kids get stronger. They are going to be incredible people, since they have had to go through this with me. There are many good, fun things that they may not have been able to experience if this hadn't happened. I will keep telling myself that.

On Thursday, Dave and I received some great news. There is a local magnet school a few blocks from our house that we had really wanted the kids to go to for school. They have a lottery system to determine if your child gets in, and families from the whole district can apply. That means kids who live close to the school like us, as well as kids who live 20+ miles away can apply. This would be great for us because it is closer to our house than the school that our kids are supposed to go to. We applied to this back in February and knew we could get picked, but we have been a bit distracted. Apparently, Alyssa's name was picked for the lottery, so she will be going to kindergarten at that elementary school starting next September. This also means that Eli will be able to attend when she is 5, so we are very excited to know that kindergarten is all lined up for both kids. Alyssa isn't sure if she is excited for elementary school, but she is very ready to be playing with kids again and really wants to start school tomorrow.

My parents took the kids for the weekend, so Dave and I enjoyed a quiet kid-free weekend. We went for a nice walk at a local park, which was great. I am limited with where we can go because I am not supposed to walk in wooded areas, so sticking to paved open paths is probably best. I prefer to walk somewhere other than in and around stores, so it was nice to find a great path with scenery. I had wanted to do the whole loop, which was 2.5 miles, but I don't even think I made it half a mile before we turned back. I found it gets a little tough to breathe with the mask on, but it really felt so good to be out in the beautiful weather. I assume the more I keep getting my strength up, the quicker I will get better. I hope to be able to do the full 2.5 miles in the coming months. We finished off the weekend with a fun trip to the farmers market in the parking lot right next door. I definitely got a lot of stares with my crazy mask, but I am getting more comfortable out in public with it, and less fazed by the random stares. Wishing you all a great week ahead!

OCTOBER 31, 2013
HAPPY HALLOWEEN FROM THE SMURFS
DAY +30

I finally have a few minutes to write an update as I just sent Dave and my mom off with Smurfette (Alyssa) and Toddler Smurf (Eli) to the mall behind our hotel to go trick or treating. I would love to join them, but an indoor space filled with children is not a good spot for me to hang out in right now, so I will just have to hear all about it when they get back. I am sad to say their costumes are pretty basic, but the felt hats I made last night seem to help define who they are. Remember how I got the bright blue leggings and shirts? They are wearing those along with hats I made for them. I took 2 pieces of white felt and cut them into the shape of a Smurf hat. I took the 2 pieces and very roughly sewed them together. Then I stuffed some paper towels into the top of it to make it look thicker. Can't you picture it? Well, it isn't our best costume ever, but it is cute. I hope that people recognize who they are dressed as. Alyssa has been so excited to go trick or treating and wear her costume (which she refused to wear half of, so hopefully people know who she is). She is also convinced that she is going to win the costume contest. I love the confidence of a four-year-old.

I am happy to say things have continued to progress smoothly. It has been 30 days since the transplant and other than the GVHD rash that has not gotten any worse, but is still present, I continue to show no other signs or complications. The doctor today told me that I should be videotaping my journey to show people how easy recovering from a transplant can be, but he then realized that it would be false advertising. I ran into my roommate from when I first arrived at Stanford, and she has had a very different experience since her transplant than I have had with mine.

I saw her at the ITA, and she was weak and looked very sick. She couldn't walk and was being pushed in a wheelchair. I couldn't believe that she was struggling so much. I now understand why my doctor was so surprised by how successful my transplant was going. It again makes me very appreciative for how lucky I have been.

My medical team has begun to make plans for my visit to the clinic around Christmas which means I will have my bone marrow biopsy and get my central line pulled before Christmas. I cannot believe this. My day 100 is supposed to be January 10, and they are talking about me going home before Christmas. I am so excited.

To make that happen, I am making sure I do everything I can to get strong. As part of my recovery, not only am I resting a lot, but I am also making sure to get plenty of exercise. I am up to about a mile a day when I can, which seems to be my max at the moment. I still hope to make it around the lake nearby, which is 2.5 miles around. Fortunately, the weather is so amazing that it has been great to be outside. In some ways, it is almost too hot. I do find exercising with the mask on is kind of hard because you can never fully catch your breath and you keep breathing in CO_2 every time, I try to take a big breath in.

It is amazing how before I went into the hospital in July I was probably in the best physical shape of my life, and now I am so weak. We are looking forward to a nice weekend with the whole family together and hopefully visiting some more of the local parks around here. I again feel so lucky to be feeling so great and getting to take advantage of this time with the family and the great weather. I can't believe I've been out of the hospital for 15 days; it feels like it has been so much longer. I look forward to hearing about everyone's weekend plans.

NOVEMBER 6, 2013
DAY +36, WHERE DOES THE TIME GO?

I can't believe it is already Wednesday night. I feel like aspects of the week go by so slowly and then next thing I know, it's been a week since I last updated everyone. I'm happy to say there is not much to update you on. Nothing to report is a good thing. My numbers continue to stay strong, and we are continuing to go to the Infusion Treatment Area (ITA) in the cancer center 2 days a week. Fortunately, I only have to be there for ~2 hours each time as all they do is draw my blood and get the results and let me go home. I have to say I much prefer this to having to get a transfusion or receive fluids or anything else. We are still working on when I will be able to get my line pulled and have my biopsy, but I am optimistic that it will be before Christmas.

The kids continue to do wonderfully. Both kids are well known throughout the hotel, Alyssa has become notorious for her chalk drawings around the sports court, and Eli is well known for greeting all the staff and guests in the dining hall. I love that both kids are so comfortable here, and I am so appreciative of the staff and how great they have been with the kids and my family. The majority of the people staying at the hotel are people who are in town for work for the week. It is nice when you see the same people. They initially stare at me, but by the end of the week they get used to me. There is another woman who is bald like me and wears knitted hats like me. There is something comforting about not being the only bald woman here. I've gotten to know her. She is also a patient at Stanford. She is waiting for her transplant. I know I complain about how far away I live, but she has got me beat. She lives on the big island of Hawaii. Isn't that incredible? She and her husband have come all the way from Hawaii for her transplant. I find it incredible that they are here for a month before they begin her transplant prep. Then she will go through the same process that I went through. It is so wonderful to not only meet a great couple but to also know someone who is going through the same thing that I am. I hope that we stay in touch.

This recent time change has done a number on all of us. The kids are starting to adjust, though Alyssa was up for the day at 5 a.m. this morning. I meanwhile find that I am falling asleep by 9 p.m. most nights. I continue to wake up twice a night to eat, which thrills the nurses and NPs at the clinic to no end. They all continue to do a double take after I let them know that I am eating constantly. I've been getting out into the community almost daily and continue to be able to tolerate odd looks (I have to admit I would stare too). I went to Costco yesterday, and there was a four-year-old boy in a cart who pointed at me from about 10 feet away and said, "What is that?" As he came closer, I told him it was my Halloween mask, and I loved it so much that I was continuing to wear it. Then I asked him if he thought it was cool. He said that he wanted to keep wearing his Halloween costume after Halloween too. Maybe I'm starting a new trend! I'm not sure how much longer I can get away with the Halloween story, but it worked.

We have a weekend of birthday celebrations here. On Friday, my grandma turns 105, and my brother turns 30 on Saturday, so I'm hoping to be able to see them both to celebrate. I look forward to hearing everyone's weekend plans.

NOVEMBER 10, 2013
WELCOME BACK DAIRY

Today is day 40 post-transplant, and I was able to start having dairy again. I am very excited to announce that I am not lactose intolerant, so dairy will become a staple again in my life. For better or worse this opens up a whole bunch of foods that I haven't been able to have since September. To celebrate, we had sparkling apple juice with dinner and homemade eggplant parmesan.

The whole family enjoyed it! We had a fabulous weekend. We broke the rules again, and on Friday went home for a few hours. It was wonderful, just nice to sit on my own couch and be in the comfort of my own home. The kids enjoyed seeing their old toys that they haven't seen in a while and playing in the backyard. We then went to my parents' house (also outside of the required safe zone) and celebrated my grandmother and brother's birthdays. We did a little family celebration and then the real party started. It was a casino-themed surprise party for my brother, and the whole living room was decorated. There were craps tables and a roulette. Cards and other decorations hung from the ceiling. It was fabulous. Alyssa really enjoyed it, and we had to pull her away from the craps table when it was time to leave. We will have to sneak her into Vegas with us. She really is good at it. I really enjoyed socializing with everyone and loved being out of the hotel for a little while. I did have to wear my mask, but I didn't care. We also had to drive the hour back to our hotel home afterwards, but that was ok. It was so much fun to get to celebrate my younger brother, the man who saved my life.

Saturday for me was a day to recover, because although I enjoyed all of the celebrating, I was tired. Apparently doing more than my basic day-to-day routine is exhausting for me. Today I had my first outing with both kids all by myself (also against the rules but worth it). There is a great farmers market in the parking lot across the street from our hotel, so I took the kids over there to get some fresh veggies and then we checked out the mall. As we went to cross the street (there aren't any crosswalks or stop signs) Alyssa asked to hold my left hand instead of my right hand. When I asked her why, she said, "So that if we get hit by a car it hits you and not me." I didn't want to point out to her that cars go in both directions. That girl cracks me up. Alyssa enjoyed pointing out everything she wants for the holidays in the mall. All was going well until Eli decided she needed to get out of the stroller and screamed the whole way home, which was probably only 5 minutes once I found my way to the door out of Macy's (which they don't make it easy to get to); it felt like an eternity. Tonight, I enjoyed watching both of my children share my love of acapella music. *Pitch Perfect* was on TV, and I called Alyssa in to enjoy the music. Eli, not wanting to miss out on anything, came running in and sat down at the base of the couch. When the singing started, Eli started dancing, clapping, and I think singing along! For better or worse this family does enjoy a good acapella mashup!

NOVEMBER 17, 2013
THE MONTH IS FLYING BY DAY +47

Can you believe it is already mid-November? I know everyone is experiencing different weather, but here in Northern California it is absolutely beautiful. Since I am somewhat confined to a hotel room and rely on good weather to be able to go out and get fresh air, I feel so lucky that we have had such great weather. It is also helpful since the kids get a chance to play outside everyday instead of being cooped up in the hotel room all day long.

I am happy to say that I continue to be boring with great numbers showing that I appear to still be leukemia free, and the GVHD rash is minimal if not almost gone. I've been waking up a lot at night lately, sometimes to eat, others just because I can't sleep, and as a result I am having lots of dreams. The other night I had a dream that I was signing up to go skydiving in January as my reward to myself for surviving the last 6 months and making it through the 100 days post-transplant. Now, before kids and marriage, I did have a slight interest in skydiving but never did it. My brother, on the other hand, has been skydiving many times. I've decided my brother's cells are taking over and starting to make some crazy choices for me. Luckily it is only in my dreams so far. When I go for my twice a week appointment at Stanford, they ask to check my ID before they draw my blood. I've had it happen 2 or 3 times now where I pull out my license and the medical assistant (who works in the cancer center) says, "Ooh, you look different with hair." It takes everything in me not to say, "Well, thank you Captain Obvious!" She really has some nerve to say that to someone in the oncology ward. Although I long to get my hair back, I've become pretty comfortable wearing hats to cover my bald head.

This week they had something I'd not seen before. It was a wig bank where they offer a complimentary wig to anyone who has become bald temporarily or permanently due to cancer.

The room had tables with many mannequin heads and mirrors. There were tons of wigs of all different colors and lengths. Now I really wanted a red or a blond wig. Wouldn't that be fun to get one that was different from how I had ever looked before? I've lived my whole life with mousy brown hair, and although I had dyed it a few times, I never went too dramatic. A wig was the perfect way to have some fun with it. Although I was tempted to try different cuts and colors, I kept getting drawn to the brown really cute bob style wig that makes me look like the old Mara. I did like that it was straight. My natural hair was always frizzy. I liked that these wigs were all straight and controlled. So if you see me with more than a few hairs on my head, chances are it is my new spicy wig. I hope to really rock the wig when I don't have to wear the huge mask along with it.

The kids continue to do great and really seem to feel at home here. Alyssa loves getting to go downstairs for breakfast and weekday dinners where she picks out exactly what she wants to eat and enjoys saying hi to the staff and other regulars. Alyssa has also recently been very interested in chapter books, so she and I are reading *Matilda* at the moment. Eli has reached 18 months and begun receiving consistent timeouts for hitting, pinching, and touching outlets. I'm not sure how effective the timeout are at the moment. She will now do any of the aforementioned defiant behaviors and then go sit over in the time out spot on her own volition. We've either done such a great job that she disciplines herself or failed miserably because she now thinks it is a game.

Hope everyone had a wonderful weekend and wishing everyone a great week ahead.

NOVEMBER 24, 2013
PASSED THE HALFWAY POINT DAY +54

Another successful yet boring week medically. This is exactly what we want; I have made it past the halfway point. I have reached day 54 today. My Monday and Thursday appointments went as smoothly as possible. My big medical drama this week is that I apparently incurred an exercise induced injury from a side plank that I did last week and had a sore shoulder for most of the week. Who would have thought that something as small and simple from a side plant could hurt me? Apparently, that is too advanced for my weak muscles; I guess I will stick with the minimal normal planks from now on. One of my nurse practitioners at the cancer center asked what I was doing for Thanksgiving, and I had to come clean and say that I would be going outside of the safe zone. She smiled and said, "I didn't hear you just say that. Have a fantastic Thanksgiving." I feel less guilty about continuously breaking the "safety zone" rules (I plan to go home at least 2 times this week).

After making a big deal last week about how nice the weather has been, we experienced our first rain of the season this week. Of course, it only lasted a day and a bit, but it was a good downpour. I was able to take advantage of something I have always wanted to do on a rainy day. I remember many rainy days at work where I would look out the window and long to be at home on the couch reading a book. I am thrilled that I was able to do just that today. I lounged on the couch, with the hotel fireplace on, and read my book looking out as the rain poured down outside. It was very relaxing and all I had ever hoped it would be. Other than the fact I was recovering from cancer, but you know what I mean.

The kids continue to be doing great. Alyssa loved jumping in puddles and checking out the worms that had all surfaced after the rain. Eli loved copying Alyssa and getting nice and dirty, fortunately she loves taking a bath, so she is easy to clean up. Both kids still seem to not be fazed by living in the hotel. Alyssa has said that she wants to move home so she can jump around and not have to have quiet feet anymore. Our hotel room is on the top floor, and I feel so bad for the people below us and our neighbors. The benefit of being on the top floor is that we don't have noisy people above us. The downfall for those below us is that we can be very loud (quick, act shocked), so we have to make sure we do not jump or stomp too loud and bother the people below us. I am just hopeful that the people around us rotate weekly and are not here for the long haul like us.

We have a big, exciting week ahead of us. Not only will we be celebrating Thanksgiving and Hanukkah at my parents' house outside of the safe zone, but it is also Dave's birthday this week. We have so much to celebrate and be thankful for. Every year at Thanksgiving we have so much to be thankful for, but this year it means so much more to us. A few months ago, we weren't sure I would even be here to celebrate. I am so grateful. We are so thankful to have all of you wonderful friends thinking about us, praying for us, and supporting us. Wishing everyone a wonderful Thanksgiving; feel free to share your Turkey Day plans.

DECEMBER 1, 2013
IMMERSED IN THE HOLIDAYS DAY +62

What a wonderful week we had; I continue to have smooth appointments, including one on Thanksgiving. Not only was it all good news, but it was also nice and quick. It only took 45 minutes from when I sat in the chair to until I walked out the door. Prior to this my quickest appointment was an hour and a half, so I certainly enjoyed the speed of this appointment. I think we were all in a hurry. The BMT doctor who was working the unit was great too; she was surprised to learn that I wasn't living back at home yet. She then said she thought I should be home in the next couple weeks. I asked her to spread the word so we could make that happen. I will keep you updated on what the new updated return home date is.

Dave enjoyed being off of work this week, so we were able to celebrate his birthday by going to a movie. In case you want to check out a new release movie without the crowd, I highly recommend the 9:45 a.m. showing on a weekday. It was great; we had perfect seats and there were maybe 30 people in a theater that could accommodate at least 400. Dave was also spoiled by a lovely buffet dinner at the hotel. I know I really do spoil him. The rest of our week was filled with appointments and celebrations. Eli had her 18-month checkup where she has gained 2 pounds since September and grown

3 inches. I'm thinking that they may have mismeasured her this time because she is in the 81st percentile for height, and Eli is quite a pipsqueak; I cannot imagine that that measurement is correct.

We had a fantastic Thanksgiving, and Alyssa led everyone in sharing what they are thankful for. She was very insistent that people go in her chosen order so we could hear them clearly. She was quite demanding, and everyone was very responsive. When it came to me, I bet you know what I was thankful for. Oh, my goodness. I am so thankful that I am still alive, thankful to my brother who saved my life, to my amazing family who helped us all trudge through these last 5 months. I truly have so much to be thankful for. Good thing Alyssa allowed me to speak clearly, and she didn't cut me off, even though I went longer than everyone else.

When we returned to our hotel home, we were surprised to see the mall parking lot behind our hotel packed as if it was a Saturday. Our location is ideal for black Friday shopping; you just have to walk across the parking lot to get to the mall.

Eli has started a new move; when you want her to do something (like give a hug) and she doesn't want to do it, instead of shaking her head no like she used to, she now pulls her arm up to her chest and sticks out her elbow. I think she looks like a matador when they do their pose. I just had an idea that maybe she has noticed I bump elbows with people instead of giving hugs, and that is why when someone asks her to give them a hug Eli pulls out the elbow. I realize I may be giving her too much credit here, but I'm going to test this theory tomorrow.

I realize I've not really mentioned this. I don't shake hands and I really don't hug anyone. I'm far less cuddly with the kids than I'd like to be. That is where the elbow touching comes into play and what Eli has turned into her new way of greeting people. Instead of shaking hands when I meet people or giving them high fives, I feel most comfortable bumping elbows. I know this looks ridiculous, but it works for me, and it makes me feel like I still am making a connection with people. Add this to the list of things I am missing so much and cannot wait to start doing again. I have found that I now have a normal appetite again; I'm not waking up in the middle of the night to eat anymore. I also find that I have more energy and don't nap during the day. I do go to sleep very early in the evening (sometimes not much later than the kids). I find my energy changes each day, and today which I am definitely more lethargic than I have been. I'm wishing everyone a wonderful week!

DECEMBER 8, 2013
BRRRRING ON THE HOLIDAYS... DAY +68

I'm happy to say that it has been another great week. Medically, things remain normal, which continues to be exactly what I want. I received great news from the attending physician in charge of the ITA. She is the doctor who had seen me on Thanksgiving and mentioned that I should be home before Christmas. Well, I saw her on Monday and asked what had to happen to achieve that goal. She said I could move home next Friday (I've never looked forward to Friday the 13th), and I only have to go to Stanford one day a week after that. We are ecstatic; all along I truly hoped that I would be home by Christmas, and when they said that I couldn't meet with my oncologist before the New Year, I had resigned myself to the fact that we would be spending Christmas and New Year's in the hotel. This is truly the best gift; well this is one of many amazing gifts (I have to give my brother and his stem cells priority here) that I have received this year.

The kids are very excited to move home, although Alyssa has said she will miss the smell of the hotel (not sure if that is a good thing). Overall, we are all ready to get home. We had a quiet weekend at the hotel with just Dave, Eli, and I. Alyssa went to Carmel with my parents for the weekend and had a blast. Alyssa is very excited to go home, but this is yet another major change for her. Ideally, it is a change back to normal (whatever that is), but she is starting to act out a bit more than she had been. When we moved into the hotel, we put up wall stickers in the kids bedroom and bathroom to make it a little more fun. When I started to take the stickers off the wall, Alyssa had a meltdown and was devastated that we were taking down her favorite stickers. Tonight, she decided to take the rest of them off by herself. I have to say she and I are very similar. We both like to be in control. I am trying to appropriately inform her as much as possible to help limit any surprises that come up along the way. Overall, I am so impressed with how both kids have handled all the changes and transitions that we have gone through over the last 6 months.

As always, I hope everyone has a great week, and for those of you in the Northern Hemisphere, stay warm.

DECEMBER 15, 2013
HOME FOR THE HOLIDAYS DAY + 75

I am so excited to be writing this update from my very own couch at my very own house. On Friday morning, we filled our car and my mom's car up with all of our remaining things at the hotel and drove back home. It really is amazing how much you can accumulate and insist you need when you will be gone for a month and a half. I mean think about it. It was a hotel, so they provided all of the kitchen stuff, the furniture, the linens, the bathroom things and more. Yet, we still had these cars full to get everything home.

I cannot explain how great it feels to be back at our house and sleeping in our bed. Since June 29, I have only spent 3 weeks and 3 nights at home. After spending almost 2 months in a hotel, I have learned that if I ever had to stay long term in a hotel again, the Homewood Suites would be my choice. Not only did they have all of the great accommodations that I was thrilled about, but the staff was so great. They were fantastic to us and always treated the kids phenomenally. Oh, according to my family, the food was pretty fantastic too.

The kids have adjusted well to being back home; Eli seems to recognize everything but also seems surprised and entertained by things she hasn't seen for 2 months. In the future when she gets bored of toys, I will just put them away for a month and then put them back out for her to play with them again like they are brand new. This will be a great way to not have to keep buying new toys. When we first came home on Friday, Alyssa ran to her room and then ran back to the front door and yelled, "Mom, my bed is not made." Clearly having housekeeping clean our room and make her bed daily spoiled her. I guess she will have to start doing it herself. We also got to bring home our dog Brady, so the whole family is officially back at home. I spent most of the weekend being a recluse, putting some things away and just laying low. I have a lot of stuff that I've been carrying around for the last 3 months that I now need to find a spot for. I actually have years of unorganized stuff that could be sorted through, so that should take me some time to keep me busy for a while. I seem to be of the mindset being home that I can now do things like I used to. I have to remember that I still need to wear my mask whenever a door or window is open, and I still have to have all my food prepared a certain way for me. There is still no eating out. I'm not sure how they came up with the rule of 100 days, but being the rule follower that I am, I will stick with what they told me.

Today is day 75, and I was able to get rid of another medication, which is definitely appreciated. On Thursday, when I went for my regular blood draw, they pulled my chest catheter out of my chest. This lets me get my future labs drawn at the local lab station through my arms like everyone else does. I am so excited, although I have learned to live with these darn lines coming out of my chest for the last 5 months, I could not wait for them to be gone. They prepped by saying that when the lines were surgically inserted, they were wrapped under my chest skin over my clavicle to be secured and then directly into my artery. Now, if you are in the medical field, this is no big deal, but to me it sounds awful. Since they said it would be an easy tug of the line, I took their word for it, and I just laid back and took a deep breath in while they tugged. It made me think of when you are pulling a chainsaw trying to get it to start. She pulled and the whole line came right out through my chest. It was crazy that this foot-long silicone tube had been in my chest for months. They said this was more difficult to pull out than they were used to because my immune system is doing so well it had already healed around the line. I now just have Steri strips and am able to take a real shower. I have to admit after 5 months of having to be so careful to not get my line wet in the shower, it is now really odd to be able to take a normal shower. That was actually the first thing I did when I got home. After the initial worry, I was very pleased to actually enjoy a warm, normal shower (it is the little things).

Think of all of the things I can do now. First thing first, I want take a real relaxing shower or a bath, instead of having to be so careful to keep the dressings dry every time I touch water. There are so many things that I used to take for granted and I can now enjoy again.

We also started to get into the holiday spirit by putting up our tree, and outdoor lights. Fortunately, we have a fake Christmas tree. We wouldn't be able to have a real one because of my potential reactions. Alyssa really enjoyed decorating the tree and carefully placed ornaments in the perfect spots. Eli seems to think that the ornaments are there for her to remove them. Many times throughout the day she excitedly brings an ornament to us off of the tree like she just found something amazing. Our tree will soon only be decorated from 32 inches and above. I also think we will hold off on putting presents below it unless we want them to all be opened early. Looking forward to a great week of continuing to get settled. Have a wonderful week.

DECEMBER 23, 2013
HO HO HOPEFUL (THIS WAS DAVE'S IDEA)
DAY +83

It is still a bit surreal that I am writing this from home, and we are going to be celebrating Christmas at home. I remember how devastated I was when I was originally reading through the transplant paperwork and realizing that I wouldn't be able to be home by Christmas. I kept hoping that I would be able to defy the odds, and so far, so good. My other wish for Christmas was that I would have hair again. Although it's not exactly the look I've been going for, it does look like my hair is all growing back and starting to fill in. One of the many side effects of this last round of chemo was that not only would I lose my hair, but I could lose it permanently. I'm glad that it decided to come on all around. Eli loves to take my hat off and massage my head.

I continue to do very well health wise. This next week is the biopsy, which is the final test to really determine how well my body has taken to the transplant and make sure there is no more leukemia in my bone marrow. It is amazing that from the biopsy they will be able to determine what percentage of my cells are my original cells versus my brother's cells. Ideally, over 95% of my cells will be my brother's. I will get all of the results on Thursday the 2nd of January when I meet with my Stanford oncologist.

While we're enjoying family time together, we have been having fun family nights out driving around the neighborhoods checking out all of the great Christmas lights. To enjoy the lights, we moved Eli's car seat forward facing for the first time. She was so enamored by finally being able to see things out the windows, she acted like the stop lights were the greatest thing she'd ever seen. Both kids (and Dave and I) love seeing everyone's decorations. We went all out tonight and went to zoo lights at the local Oakland Zoo. It was very fun, and we all enjoyed the decorations. This was the first kid focused venue I have been to since wearing the mask. Fortunately, it was dark while we were walking around, so I avoided a lot of stares. I also learned that I can put my scarf over my mask and I just look like I am ready for a much colder climate. The highlight of the evening was that there was a Santa Claus there, and Eli sat on his lap while Alyssa stood at the base of the sled. This is impressive, since Alyssa usually runs the other way if she even hears Santa is in the general vicinity. This is the first Santa picture I have of the kids since Alyssa was 9 months old. Alyssa said she was happy she was able to be in the picture, but she would not be getting any closer to Santa in the future. That's my girl. Wishing everyone a wonderful week of family and celebrations.

DECEMBER 30, 2013
BRING ON 2014! DAY +90

What a wonderful week of celebrating with family and friends. I truly enjoyed so much of this past week. We had a wonderful time as a family on Christmas Eve and got to carry on some traditions from my childhood, like reading "'Twas The Night Before Christmas" and other holiday favorites. It was wonderful to see the kids enjoying Christmas. Of course, Eli is at the age where the box that a gift comes in is played with more than the toy itself, but she managed to play with all of her new goodies. Alyssa also enjoyed her gifts and surprised us all by being so appreciative and thankful to everyone for her gifts. It is really so amazing for me to watch Alyssa try on different phrases and attitudes to see how people respond. Don't get me wrong; some of these absolutely infuriate me, but she truly is testing to see what types of responses she gets when she acts different ways and says different things. Eli has recently begun using the word "Ow" as her primary vocab word. I wasn't sure why she said it so often until I realized it is the word she hears most often as she goes up to her sister and pinches her or pulls her hair. She also is a bit of a klutz and often bumps her head or falls down. She also likes to give out a warning by announcing "ow" right before she pinches you. Alyssa definitely takes the brunt of her abuse because she is the only one with hair long enough to pull.

I had another successful appointment and was thrilled when I found out that my bone marrow biopsy on Thursday was only an aspiration. The last 3 times they have done both the aspiration and taken out bits of bone, so I was thrilled to not have to have the bone part biopsied too. I go in on the 2nd to get the official results and learn more about how things will be able to move forward, since I'm almost at day 100. They continue to discontinue many of my medications, which is great. The only problem I have learned is that by discontinuing those medications I have to increase my immune suppressant medications. Unfortunately, the increase has caused me the most discomfort I have had throughout this whole process.

On Friday and Saturday, I spent much of the day in bed fighting off a headache and stomachache. Fortunately, thanks to Tums and a new medication that seems to have finally kicked in, I am a lot more comfortable. I have to say it was a bit daunting to have done so well through this whole process to then be so uncomfortable due to something as simple as a basic medication. Fingers crossed they don't have to keep increasing my immunosuppressants.

We are looking forward to a quiet and celebratory New Year's Eve (I may be celebrating the east coast New Years since the chances of me staying up until midnight are slim to nil).

Here's to a fabulous New Year to everyone filled with health and happiness.

JANUARY 7, 2014
WELCOME 2014 HAPPY 2014 DAY +98

I hope everyone was able to bring in the New Year with friends, family, and a great evening. I was shocked to have actually stayed up until 12:45 a.m. 2014, which was pretty impressive, since I can barely stay up until 10 p.m. most nights. The year 2013 was certainly a doozy, and I hope the worst year of my life. I'm looking forward to a great year. So far, 7 days in, the year has delivered wonderfully!

On January 2, I went to see my oncologist at Stanford. This was the very first doctor that I met at Stanford, and he is the one who told me about the SCT and got me set up to be admitted to Stanford. I then did not see him again for 4 months. The reason I never saw him for these 4 months is because the doctors that see you in the hospital are only the on-call doctors. The doctors are on call for a month at a time, so he was not on call during these last few months. I was so happy I got to see him again. He was very pleased with how well I have been doing. With that, he brought in a dose of reality. He reminded me that I have no immune system and not begun to produce T-Cells. Those are part of the immune system that develop from stem cells. That is why even though these first 100 days have been so successful, I still have to be so careful when out and about.

I had thought that at this time I would have the immune system of a newborn baby, but apparently, I have not even begun to produce new cells, and I probably won't for another 3 months. Therefore, I need to continue to be very careful with what I am around. I will go back to see him in 2 weeks and learn about what percentage of my cells are Ben's versus mine.

Due to the holidays, they had not yet completed determining that portion of the results. What they had been able to see was that my cells currently showed that I am still in remission, which is wonderful. In addition, my numbers continue to look good. My extreme stomach pain is supposedly just indigestion, so I have new meds to coat my stomach, and I was told that I should take Tums for more immediate relief. I also got cleared to drive myself, cook for myself (which I had been doing anyway), and go out in public without my mask on (unless I'm at a construction site or a medical clinic). I want to take a minute to fully appreciate all of this. I know for him this is just the basic thing he tells patients. I'm sure for you this sounds like another basic thing. However, I really need to take a minute to really appreciate what this means. For over 100 days I have not been able to drive ANYWHERE by myself. I have had to rely on other people for EVERYTHING. Since I couldn't just order food to be delivered, I would need to get food from the store, since I couldn't drive, I would need someone to get me to the store or get the food for me. Then it would need to be cooked. Since I wasn't supposed to cook myself (although sometimes I did) I would need someone else to cook it for me. Are you seeing here how annoying this is?

Hearing my doctor lift all these restrictions and give me this independence made me feel amazing. Once again, I hadn't realized how held back I had been feeling. That means that for the first time in more than 100 days I can feel independent again. I know there were a few days since June 30 I was able to run errands, but there were very few. What did I want to do now that I had this newfound freedom? I am now going to run errands by myself and drive myself wherever I want to go.

The kids continue to thrive. I am so lucky to get to spend so much time with them. Back when I used to work all of the time, I was spending all day working and barely getting to spend time with the kids until the evenings. I love that now my time is all theirs. We were all home as a family for the last 2 weeks, which was great. Dave went back to work today, and the kids were back with a new caregiver during the day so I could rest and go to appointments. They are so good at acclimating to new situations. Eli has begun to have a little bit of separation anxiety. I'm not sure if it is because she misses us or because she feels left out. This morning when Dave left and I was still with Eli, she cried and cried, wanting to be with Dave. Luckily, she calms down easily too, but this is really the first separation anxiety we've seen out of her. Alyssa had her first sleepover at a friend's house this weekend, and it went well. Dave and I are already planning date nights for when both kids are doing sleepovers. Last week I mentioned that Alyssa was trying out new sayings. This week her response to anything that she doesn't understand is: "Blah, blah, blah" and "Vice versa." I'm still working on helping her use *vice versa* appropriately, but until then I will enjoy her silly sayings.

I'm looking forward to hearing about everyone's start to 2014!

JANUARY 16, 2014
KEEP THE GOOD NEWS COMING

Today was another first; I was able to drive myself to my appointment at Standford for the first time since September. I love the sense of freedom of being able to drive myself, even if it takes 4 hours round trip. Today was much quicker than last time (it helps to be the first patient of the day). Everything still looks good, and my next appointment will be in 3 weeks when we will start tapering down my immunosuppressant medication. I completely forgot to ask about what percentage of my cells are mine versus Ben's, so I'll email to ask about that and have the info by next week.

I have been freaking out a bit this week about the H1N1 virus, as well as the stomach bug that is going around. I'm finding that I often have to pass on social situations to avoid any chance of catching anything. The guidelines they have given me say that I can do everything without my mask on, including attending concerts, movies, sporting events, etc. However today when I told my doctor that I wear a mask at Costco, and that's where I get the craziest stares, his response was, "Costco. Mara, there are a lot of people there. You shouldn't be around that many people." Basically, I'm realizing that I really should lay low.

I was going to bring up a foot injury to Dr. M, my Stanford doctor, today. The top of my left foot has been hurting for the last week, and I was afraid there was something going on that I should be worried about. Fortunately, this morning I realized as I shoved my foot into my tennis shoe without untying it, that my foot probably hurts because I don't put my shoes on in a conventional manner. Wouldn't that be the reason my foot is hurting and not some bigger reason? I'll try untying and tying my shoes like a normal person for a week or so, and then if I'm still uncomfortable I'll bring it up to my doctor.

While I am hanging out at home, one of my big goals is to get the house somewhat organized. I see I'm constantly trying to organize my house. Not to get too psychological, but I think there is a much bigger issue here with the fact that so much of my life is out of control and cleaning/organizing my house is the only thing within my control. Look, I just saved time and money by not needing to visit a psychologist. Before June, I always felt that I was struggling to keep up with tidying up our house; now I finally have time. After being home for a month, I finally emptied and put away the final 3 suitcases worth of stuff that I had at the hospital and hotel. I am also going through the kids' rooms and feeling quite a sense of accomplishment as I make some headway. It helps that the kids are out of the house during the day, so they aren't pulling out everything that I'm putting away. Alyssa appears to have been a Depression-Era hoarder in a previous life. The other day she had brought home some plastic to-go containers and cleaned them out so she could store things in them. I have to wait for her to leave for the day and systematically throw things away that she has collected, including all of the Penny Savers and other ads we get in the mail. Eli has begun talking a lot more in the last week or two, which has been fun. We still don't understand it all, but she is quite vocal, and occasionally we are quite impressed with ourselves when we can understand what she says. To make sure she keeps getting attention, Eli has been eating like crazy, waking up in the middle of the night more, and on the less fun side of things, she has begun biting. I remember Alyssa went through a very fast biting stage, so I am hoping this will be quick also. I am a bit nervous, though, because whenever we discipline her, she just looks at us and laughs. We may be in for it with her. Dave and I are looking forward to a date night this weekend. Who knows? Maybe we'll be able to stay out and awake until 8 p.m. or 9 p.m.; we are living on the wild side lately.

JANUARY 28, 2014
WAIT FOR IT... SO IT IS OFFICIAL

I am now 97% my brother. Yes, 97% of my cells are Ben's, and they consider anything over 95% full chimerism. Chimerism is my vocab word of the month. You may have heard of this in mythological terms. You know the monster who is the head of a goat and the body of a lion? Well, this is also a term that they use with humans when the person has cells from 2 different sources. Isn't that strange? I'm not huge into mythology and also not huge into science, but I do love mystery stories, so here is what really helped me understand this. So, get this. If I ever commit a crime and leave blood at the scene, they would never suspect me. Isn't that wild? You see, since the blood I am producing is predominantly my donor's (my brother) DNA, then they would be searching for a male not female. And my brother's DNA so they wouldn't suspect me. Isn't that wild? Now I'm not out to commit a crime, but I'm just saying... Sorry, Ben.

Yesterday, I joined the Cancer Support Community (CSC), which is a center that helps people impacted with cancer by providing support throughout their cancer journey. This is the only one in the Bay Area, and it happens to be less than a mile from my house. Remember how when I was in the hospital, I wanted to create a group of those of us going through the same thing? Well, this is exactly what this CSC provides. I learned about this place when I was first diagnosed, but since I was always in the hospital or far away, I was never able to attend their many great programs. I've always known that this would be a good environment for me, since everyone has a suppressed immune system, and their goal is to help cancer patients and their caregivers either during or post treatment. I am looking forward to meeting other people on this journey. At the same time, I am nervous about whether or not I can be part of a group without taking on other people's challenges as my own. I am sure this is something all of these people struggle with. I know I will share more with you here as I learn more.

This last week I was introduced to a woman who was diagnosed with a different type of leukemia in July. She will be undergoing a BMT in the next couple months and is experiencing a lot of the anxiety that I experienced prior to my transplant. I am so glad that I am available to support her. It feels so wonderful to be able to share my experience and give her strength and comfort as she faces this journey. I remember feeling the same anxiety she is experiencing and am glad that I already went through the transplant and 100 days afterwards. I know I am only 3 months post-transplant, but I feel like I am such an expert. I hope I can offer comfort to this other patient as she prepares.

On a lighter note, things are going very well on the home front. We are getting into a routine, or as much of one as we can. Dave and the kids went to the zoo this last weekend. Eli ran around and enjoyed the animals. Also, today Dave turned in all of the paperwork for Alyssa to be enrolled into the magnet kindergarten that is very close to our house. I can't believe she's almost in school. Eli's language is growing. She does have a handful of words that we understand and quite a few that we don't understand at all. It's so funny when she goes off on these long gibberish sentences with great intonation, etc. She's also eating like crazy, and she seems to be really gaining weight. It's kind of hard for me to tell, but I definitely notice it when I have to hold her for a while. I guess I don't have to exercise; I can just carry her around to get my strength training in.

Although most of my rule-breaking days are done, I have been breaking a few rules. These are the rules that I wanted to follow only because I didn't want to do the tasks. I have been changing Eli's dirty diapers, which was a no-no, and also picking up after Brady (the dog). For diapers and picking up after Brady, I wear latex gloves. I was feeling guilty going for walks and leaving poor Brady at home, so he now comes along with me as we tour our great neighborhood.

FEBRUARY 19, 2014
TRUDGING ALONG

I can't believe it has been just over 3 weeks since my last post. I guess that is a great indicator that things are feeling like they are getting back to normal. I have continued to do well and had another appointment with Dr. M at Stanford last Thursday. We started reducing my immunosuppressant medication, which we will do gradually over the next couple months. We only reduce 1mg per day every 2 weeks (and I started on 8 mgs a day), so it will take until May before I am off all of the immunosuppressants as long as things go smoothly. So far, I've been down to 7 mgs a day for a week and had no GVHD appear yet, so I'm optimistic that this slow tapering will help reduce any GVHD issues. On Friday, I started to have symptoms similar to allergies, and when I contacted my doctor, he felt that since there had been a lot of repertory infections this year, he started me on Tamiflu and a Z-Pack, an antibiotic just to make sure I don't have beginning symptoms of the flu. I feel fine now, and the whole family is putting up with the sniffles. I have been keeping myself busy with a couple yoga classes a week at CSC, and I also attend a weekly support group which has been both difficult and rewarding. The group is made up to 15 people with different types of cancer. Since the group is early in the day, it is mostly retired older people and a few who are currently out of work on disability. Everyone has different types of cancers and are at different stages of their treatment. I am the only one who is in remission, which makes me feel that I stand out. Standing out in a good way is not a bad thing at all. With that, I know that this is still very important for me to be here. I have had very little interaction with other cancer patients, and I need to talk to people who understand what I am going through but are not emotionally attached to me. I am so appreciative of my family and friends, but at the same time I want to stay strong for them, and I know they are trying to stay strong for me. At home, everyone is so positive, which is fantastic and a major part of what is keeping me going. In this group, people are very open and realistic. They share their experience, where they are in their treatments. Things that have helped them, as well as things that have not. Different foods, natural products, doctors, insurance advice, and studies they know about. This group is a wealth of information from people who are going through the same thing I am. This group is also a place where I can be open and share things that I didn't even know I was holding onto. I felt comfortable crying openly with these strangers because they do not judge me, and they understand what I am going through.

One woman in the group is a bit older than me. She has 3 daughters, one age 10 and twins who are 13. She came into the group the first time I met her. She was carrying 3 boxing gloves. When she introduced herself, she said that she was just diagnosed with breast cancer for the third time, and she was going to fight, but she was getting tired. I couldn't help putting myself in her shoes. She is so impressive fighting this fight. She talked about what if she didn't make it through this third fight. For the first time in these last 7 months I thought, *Oh crap, what if I hadn't made it through?* I could have died. I am so lucky to be in remission, and thanks to the SCT, I will be cancer free forever. I am so lucky.

This organization CSC and all that they offer mentally and physically is a lifesaver for me.

The kids have been doing really well. I got to take Alyssa to the new Lego movie as a special mommy and daughter day. It has been fun to have special time just the two of us. Alyssa has been doing tons of artwork and is loving practicing letters and numbers all day long. One of her other favorite activities is going through our recycle bin and taking everything out to use it for a craft project. Now I love that she is interested in upcycling and reusing things, but I have to admit that her need to be pulling things out of the recycle and spreading it around our house is not something I'm a big fan of. I find that the more that I try to clean up the house, the more the kids feel the need to pull everything out all over the place. Speaking of little disasters, Eli is definitely a little "Wreck it Ralph." She feels most comfortable in an environment where everything is all over the floor all around her. She is also starting to be more and more self-sufficient. The other day she was in the front room, and I was watching from a distance. She climbed up into her highchair and pulled the tablecloth towards her so she could reach a piece of cake that was in the middle of the table. I have to say I was pretty impressed that she was able to do that herself.

I find that I'm really trying to make the most of my time with the kids when I can. With that being said, sometimes I have to remind myself that when the kids are acting crazy, or just driving me crazy, I am just lucky to be here to experience this.

I continue to appreciate and thrive from all of your prayers and positive thoughts. I look forward to hearing from you and what you and your family have been up to.

MARCH 16, 2014
BIRTHDAYS AND MOVIES

Today is a very special day. Today is Alyssa's birthday, and I am so happy to get to celebrate her birthday with her as a family all at home together and feeling really good. This is one of the many reasons why I went through all the chemo, the transplant, and everything to keep me alive. I did this so I could be here for all of these wonderful celebrations. Eli seems to be enjoying Alyssa's birthday almost as much as she is.

In other fun news, control your excitement, but you now know 4 movie stars. Yes, I too am shocked, but the Solomon family has been asked to be in a short documentary-style video. Now this may not get nominated for an Oscar, or even presented at Sundance, but a film is being made about the Stanford bone marrow transplant nurses, and they have asked us to be in a part of the video. I'm not sure yet if this is used for training purposes or to be available to people as a patient education film. Regardless, I am excited that they have chosen to work with us as one of the families who have been through the transplant process. They actually just called me about the shoot while I was writing this. Alyssa is excited about her moment on film. We are choosing our outfits.

I had another appointment with my transplant oncologist last week, and he continues to be pleased with how things are going. I continue to reduce the Prograf (immune suppressant medication) every other week with very minimal GVHD. He also let me know that although they often do a bone marrow biopsy at 6 months post-transplant, he does not find it necessary to do it for me. If they did the biopsy and there were leukemic cells present (which there should not be), they would have to reduce my Prograf and do a round of chemo, as well as another transplant of sort. Long story short, since my numbers remain stable, there is no reason to believe that there is any return of the leukemia, and therefore I have decided not to have the biopsy next month.

I find that I have been getting very achy at the end of the day, which is a result of reducing my immune suppression medication. I'm usually okay during the day, but at night if I've been sitting for a bit, it takes me a minute to get up, and I move a bit slower. Otherwise, I'm getting more and more energy back, and my hair is long enough that I can feel comfortable going out without a hat. Now let me clarify "long enough." I basically have what looks like a buzz cut. That is how long my hair is now, which is great. The fact that my hair is growing back at all is great. I love that it is even brown with now gray, and it is growing out evenly all around my head. Watch out; I may have to shave my head along with Dave soon.

In the past couple weeks, Dave has had to occasionally work late, and I've handled the evening and bedtime routine on my own. It makes me continue to be in awe of what an amazing job Dave did while I was in the hospital. I can't believe he did all that he did for 3 months while working full time and having to worry about what was going on with me. He is well on his way to dad of year! We're looking forward to another week of wonderful weather and our video shoot this weekend. I can't wait to tell you all about it.

APRIL 1, 2014
6 MONTHS POST-TRANSPLANT, 9 MONTHS INITIAL DIAGNOSIS

This is not an April Fool's joke. Today is officially 6 months since I had my stem cell transplant, and tomorrow will mark 9 months since my original diagnosis of leukemia. WOW! I am so excited to be able to report that things continue to go very well, and I have made it to another milestone in my road to recovery. I continue to feel really good, minus a few aches due to reducing my immune suppressant. Overall, the indigestion/stomach aches are gone, thanks to medication and the occasional Tums. I am continuing to deal with a very minimal case of GVHD, which represents itself in dry skin and a barely noticeable rash on my neck. I consider myself very lucky to have such a minimal case of it. Even though it is minimal, it is still very painful. Since skin is the largest organ in the human body, it is no surprise that it is being affected by this transplant. For the dry rash, it is especially on my torso and feels like a constant itch all over my body. You know when you have that itch that you just can't scratch? That is what it feels like, and it is off and on all day long. I am lucky many times that I can sleep through it, but as soon as I rub it against something, either by mistake or on purpose, then the itch starts up again. I have been given some steroid cream. I hope it helps. It is a really gross, clear Vaseline-like ointment. Like I say, it better help because I don't want this whole process to be for nothing. I hope to be off of all of the immune suppressants in 6 weeks, when we should have a good idea of how aggressive the GVHD will be when the new cells are no longer being suppressed.

I still am very cautious when I go out. I remain a bit of a recluse but love that I'm able to be with my family and enjoy the craziness that is my life. We have had a fun couple of weeks planned exploring with both kids, continuing to let their personalities grow and shine. Like most of America and possibly the rest of the world, our household is obsessed with the *Frozen* soundtrack. So much so that Eli requests the "With You" song every time we get into the car. Another musical that we are focusing on is *The Sound of Music*. Alyssa starts a new theater class shortly. This is the first time since September that we are letting her go to a group class due to our hypersensitivity to germs this year. I am sure she will have a blast and hope that most of this year's contagious illnesses are not able to affect her.

A few weeks ago, the kids and I had to pick up a prescription at Kaiser, and while we were waiting for it, we went up to the third floor to visit the nurses who were so awesome to me while I was there. It was great to get to check in with them and see them again. Visiting them by choice and while I was healthy was so fun. One of the nurses was pregnant now. She wasn't pregnant 9 months ago when I was on the floor. Shoot, I remember learning all about the man she loved so much and all of the fun she was. How fun to see her now. It was really great to see how all of our lives have moved forward. In our cases it has moved along for the better. These nurses were such an integral part in my journey. I was of course sporting my awesome HEPA filter mask; I look forward to being able to go back and visit without the mask.

We had the pleasure this last week of rebooking our Hawaiian vacation that we had to cancel last year. It felt great to get to book the trip again. Having something to look forward to is so important. It's not for 8 months or so, but it is nice to have something to look forward to. I also had a wonderful rep at Alaska Airlines who I dealt with. She was great; not only was she so helpful, but she also waived the $300 change fees for our tickets. It might not be much, but it meant a lot to me. There have been many of these things and I really have a new way of looking at them.

Dave and Alyssa had the opportunity to go to Sacramento last week to watch the school Dave works at play for the boys' Basketball Division State Championship. It was at the King's arena, and Dave's school won. Alyssa and Dave (who made it on TV) had a great time. Alyssa's memorable moments from the game involve eating candy and watching the cheerleaders, and even though they were only a few rows from the court, I'm not sure that she watched any of the actual basketball, but she had a great time. I hope you are enjoying spring's recent emergence in most parts of the country. I look forward to hearing how you are doing.

MAY 1, 2014
LONG TIME NO UPDATE

I can't believe it has been a month since my last post. In my case, no news is actually good news. Things have continued to go wonderfully. At my last doctor's appointment, my transplant oncologist was very pleased with how things have gone over the last 6 months. I still have to be careful, but he had me schedule my next appointment for 8 weeks out. He said making it past 6 months was a big milestone, with 9 months being my next one.

I continue to taper down my immunosuppressant medications and should be off of them in 2 weeks. That means that once I am off them, I should have the immune system of an unvaccinated 6-month-old. I have been concerned that I have super dry skin on my face and scalp that is a sign of GVHD. My doctor was not impressed and said to just put lotion on and to use some Selsun Blue, an over-the-counter cream, on the dry spots if I am concerned. He continues to remind me that these very mild signs of GVHD continue to be a good sign and that I should be able to easily take care of this. It is really nice to know that some of the things that I think are big concerns seem to be no big deal.

A couple weeks ago, during Dave's spring break we got to go on a road trip to Southern California. It was fantastic. It was so nice to physically and emotionally get away. The kids did great on the drive, and for the first time we truly felt like we could live life again. I still had to be super careful about germs, and we didn't visit any theme parks or anything, but that didn't stop us from enjoying everything we could. I enjoyed walking on the beach, and I think I look like a movie star trying to go unnoticed, because I have my hat, sunglasses, and hooded sweatshirt on.

The kids continue to grow; Eli was so proud of herself tonight as she was able to put her own pajama pants on. She also loves to dress up as a princess and call herself Princess Elsa (how she says Eli). Alyssa is loving her theater class. She was assigned the part of Liesl in the *Sound of Music*. She has a few lines and sings 2 stanzas of "I Am 16 Going on 17." It is very fun to watch her practice her lines, and a bit scary when she sings the song because she truly acts and thinks she is 16 going on 17.

I find that I am frequently talking about the village of friends and family that have supported us through the last 10 months, and how valuable you are to us. Have a wonderful Friday and weekend.

JUNE 6, 2014
SUMMER IS HERE

Another month and a bit has gone by, and things continue to move forward in a positive direction. We celebrated Eli's 2nd Birthday a couple weeks ago, which is so unbelievable. I can't believe she is 2. She loved when people said "Happy Birthday" to her and would often respond with an exuberant "Happy Birthday." She also blew out her own candle with just a little bit of help. She has enjoyed singing "Happy Birthday" regularly to many people whenever she feels the urge. My health continues to improve.

I am at the lowest possible dose of immunosuppressant, which is .5 mg once a day. I have begun to have some arthritis-like symptoms in my hands that are more of an inconvenience than anything. I saw the doctor at Stanford yesterday; he says the joint pain is exactly what I should be feeling as I reduce the meds. I just need to be patient, as I will be off the immune suppressants next Wednesday. It helps me to know that the pain and discomfort is a sign of reducing the meds and not something else. In the back of my mind, I keep thinking that every ailment, pain, and more is a sign of the cancer coming back. This is the most important time to keep an eye on any increasing GVHD issues.

As of June 1, I am 8 months post-transplant, which is so exciting. I was just informed at my appointment that lots of chronic GVHD does not become apparent until 9 months post-transplant. I hope that I am part of the 25% of sibling transplant recipients that have no chronic GVHD and whatever I am experiencing is just very mild to nonexistent GVHD.

One of the things I am doing to keep myself busy lately is organizing and going through things. I know I keep saying that, but I really am working on it. I enjoy collecting and saving things and have recently come across a box of things that I have saved from high school, college, and beyond. As I was going through things, I found a parking ticket that I had saved. Saving this was even a bit much for me, so I went to throw it out and saw that there was a letter attached to it. Turns out I had received the parking ticket when I was parked at UC Berkeley while helping run a bone marrow donor sign up to get more people nationally registered. These random reminders of how involved bone marrow registration has been in my life. if my brother hadn't been a match, I would have relied on that list to find a donor and hopefully find a match.

Alyssa is looking forward to her *Sound of Music* production. She has her lines and song pretty much memorized, and we continue to practice them with her. I have to say I have always been a fan of the song "16 Going on 17" but never knew the lyrics like I do now. The following is what Alyssa at the age of 5 will be singing and acting.

She will be playing the role of a 16-year-old singing this:

"I am 16 going on 17. I know that I'm naïve. Fellows I meet may tell me I'm sweet, and willingly I believe. I am 16 going on 17, innocent as a rose. Bachelor dandy, drinkers of brandy, what do I know of those? Totally unprepared am I, to face the world of men. Timid and shy and scared am I of things beyond my ken. I need someone older and wiser, telling me what to do. I am 16, going on 17. I depend on you."

The words are quite interesting, and slightly disturbing. I look forward to getting a video of this not only to share, but also to show her when she is 16.

The school year is finishing up for Dave, and we are looking forward to a summer together as a family. I can't wait to see what adventures lie ahead of us. I would love to hear what adventures you have coming up this summer.

JUNE 12, 2014
WE ARE FAMOUS

Remember a few months ago when I told you that the Solomons were going to be movie stars? Well, the movie debuted today, and I have the link. The video is part of the Stanford Hospital and Clinics Pride series. This one focuses on the E1 unit nurses, which is where they do all of the bone marrow and stem cell transplants. ENJOY!

http://www.youtube.com/watch?v=ILNIgiBll34

Have a fabulous weekend.

JUNE 29, 2014
WHAT A YEAR

One year ago, today Dave drove me to the ER to be admitted for what we were really hoping was just some fluke illness. As we all now know, things turned out to be much more serious than I could have ever imagined. With all of the drama that we have had to endure, we are so grateful that everything is okay.

To celebrate, we spent this last weekend camping a few hours from home with just our family. It reminded me that the last camping trip we went on in 2013 was the weekend before I went into the hospital. Which made the trip this weekend feel like I was heading back into normalcy. It really is full circle. This is how our life will be. We are going to live it to the fullest because we have had to learn how important it is to not take anything for granted.

RESOURCES

American Cancer Society is a leading organization that works to end cancer by providing support and guidance to people affected by cancer. cancer.org

Be the Match is an international organization that matches donors with patients from around the world. BeTheMatch.org

Cancer Support Community is a national organization that provides services for people and their family as they live or have lived with cancer. Cancersupport.com

Leukemia & Lymphoma Society is the largest nonprofit dedicated to creating a world without blood cancers. lls.org

ACKNOWLEDGEMENTS

I want to take a moment here to thank all of the amazing people who have stood by me during this incredibly challenging time in my life. First and foremost, my husband, Dave Solomon, and my kids, Alyssa and Eli Solomon. You are my everything, you are the reason I kept pushing through every challenge along the way. You are the light at the end of the tunnel and the reason I insisted on fighting so hard to make it through. You also supported me as I made this book a reality.

My brother Ben Rothman. It is thanks to you that I am alive. Thank you for sharing your stem cells to keep me alive. You didn't have to do it, but you did, and it is thanks to you that I am alive today.

Thank you to my parents, Al and Arlyss Rothman, who stood by my side and helped bring some normalcy to this extremely challenging situation so we could all keep living life through this out-of-control life. You always stepped in to watch the kids, be my caregiver, and so much more. Your great tips, connections and advocating for me helped my pull through. Watching your strength as you faced this disease so well became a model for my own journey.

I am beyond thankful for my village near and far, you all know who you are. Those of you who supported me and my whole family throughout this journey. You brought food, walked the dog, watched the kids. You said prayers, sent cards, gifts, emails, calls, visits. You offered advice, told jokes, gave me words of encouragement, and ways to be distracted. I am thankful for all of you for holding me and my family together to help us get through everything.

My medical team the doctors and nurses on the third floor Kaiser Walnut Creek and the E1 unit and the ITA at Stanford Hospital who helped get me through a terrifying time.

Thank you to Stephanie Feger at the emPower PR Group for guiding me through every step of this journey. You helped me turn this book idea into a reality. I knew what I wanted to do but didn't know all that it required to make it a reality. Thank you for connecting me with an incredible editing team—and an amazing art and design team—who created the cover, imprint, and more. Your ideas and execution are beautiful.

ABOUT THE AUTHOR

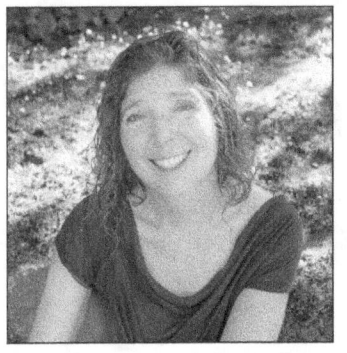 Mara Solomon is a cancer survivor, who has dedicated her life to help people live their life to the fullest. She is making sure that cancer will not bring her down and encourages other people who are faced with cancer and other health challenges do the same.

As a married mother of two beautiful daughters, she spends her time staying healthy, traveling, and living life to the fullest. Her motto is: Do what you can, where you can, when you can.

You can learn more about Mara and all of the incredible resources she uses and shares with people whose lives have been affected by cancer on her website at LivingLifeAfterCancer.com.

www.ingramcontent.com/pod-product-compliance
Lightning Source LLC
Chambersburg PA
CBHW061552120626
46550CB00004B/1455